Working with Relationship Triangles

The Guilford Family Therapy Series
Michael P. Nichols, *Series Editor*

Working with Relationship Triangles

The One-Two-Three of Psychotherapy

Philip J. Guerin, Jr.
Thomas F. Fogarty
Leo F. Fay
Judith Gilbert Kautto

Series Editor's Note by Michael P. Nichols

THE GUILFORD PRESS
New York London

©1996 The Guilford Press
A Division of Guilford Publications, Inc.
72 Spring Street, New York, NY 10012
www.guilford.com

Printed in the United States of America

This book is printed on acid-free paper.

Last digit is print number: 9 8

Library of Congress Cataloging-in-Publication Data

Working with relationship triangles : the one-two-three
of psychotherapy / Philip J. Guerin, Jr. ... [et al.].
    p.   cm. — (The Guilford family therapy series)
    Includes bibliographical references and index.
    ISBN 978-1-60623-917-9 (paperback)
    ISBN 978-1-57230-143-6 (hardcover)
    1. Triangles (Interpersonal
relations) 2. Psychotherapy.
    3. Group psychotherapy. I. Guerin, Philip J.,
Jr. II. Series.
    RC489.T82W67 1996
    616.89′14—dc20   96-33339
                                                   CIP

In memory of Murray Bowen

Series Editor's Note

Having begun competitive weightlifting in my middle years, I discovered the need for stretching the hard way. I'd pull various muscles and then realize—*Oh, I should have been stretching that!* As a therapist, I discovered triangles much the same way. I'd try something reasonable with the people in the consulting room, but sometimes it wouldn't go well. *Oh, I should have taken into account the live-in boyfriend or grandmother*—the third party who hadn't even been mentioned before.

Some triangles are obvious—the extramarital affair, the parents who don't agree about how to treat their problem child. In these familiar cases, most of us eventually learn that the presenting problem isn't going to improve until the triangular complications are dealt with.

For many of us, that's the extent of our knowledge of triangles—that they sometimes complicate things and that in those cases they must be worked out somehow. How wonderful, then, to come across this book by Phil Guerin and his colleagues with its rich, systematic analysis of triangles and how to resolve them. A knowledge of triangles, as the authors say, can sometimes produce amazing results. In *Working with Relationship Triangles*, Guerin, Fogarty, Fay, and Kautto don't just make that claim, they back it up with a wealth of detailed explanation about a whole variety of triangles—and how to treat them.

So, how relevant is a book about relationship triangles in the quick-fix era of managed care?

You might think that exploring relationship triangles is relevant only to long-term, intensive therapies. Nothing could be further from the truth. A brief therapist who intervenes aggressively may achieve temporary progress, but if important triangles aren't dealt with, this progress may not last. Uncovering triangles, on the other hand, can often lead to immediate and fundamental changes in the functioning of a relationship system. For anyone working with family problems, thinking about triangles helps keep the focus on the structural problems and avoid being recruited into the role of trying to solve a family's problems for them.

The very first family I treated was a good example. "Tito Ramirez" was a 5-year-old boy who set fire to his family's apartment. When I interviewed Tito and his young mother and 3-year-old sister, all I saw was a quiet boy, a rambunctious 3-year-old, and a distracted mother. Only when I shut up and listened to the mother long enough to hear that her primary preoccupation was problems with her boyfriend, did I recognize the triangle that was at the root of the little firesetter's unhappiness. Although I had no knowledge of family dynamics, I had enough common sense to realize that the number-one priority in Ms. Ramirez's life was working things out with her boyfriend. Once she did that—it took about two sessions—and had some security and a little love in her life, she was able to turn her attention to her children.

While it may be that family systems therapists are more likely than others to understand triangles, the importance of uncovering relationship triangles isn't limited to any particular approach. Even individual therapists, as the authors explain, often bog down in stalemated treatments due to unresolved triangles. In this marvelously useful guide, they show how coaching individuals can help resolve triangles, and they explain when and how to bring other members of the triangle into treatment. If someone were to make a list of the ten most useful books ever written about family systems, *Working with Relationship Triangles* would surely make the list.

MICHAEL P. NICHOLS
Williamsburg, Virginia

Preface

This book is about thinking in threes—in our own families and in our clinical work—about what we'll find if we think in threes and about what to do when we find it. Since the days of Freud, many rich and useful languages have developed for thinking about the individual: psychoanalysis, object relations theory, and behaviorism among them. Many of these languages have been equally rich and useful for thinking about dyads. Murray Bowen and some of the other founders of family systems theory thought it was significant that people often organized their interior lives and their relationship lives in threes (e.g., mom, dad, and me; me, my best friend, and my friend's best friend; me, my spouse, and my child). Bowen, especially, tried to develop a new language—one which would help us think and talk about these triangles.

Like any new language, this one is still in its youth, and so it's nowhere as mature as earlier psychological and psychiatric languages. We hope this work moves the language of threes a little further along. That's what we wanted to do when we decided to write this book. Our experience in our own lives and with patients has convinced us of the usefulness of "thinking triangles" for figuring out people, relationships, families, and other human social systems. But talking to other therapists about triangles, our own difficulties in formulating ideas about them, and the different ways therapists approach the idea, led us to believe that the idea of triangles was less than completely worked out. There was a lack of sharpness in our own and others' understanding of triangles, and sometimes different therapists seemed to be talking about different things when they spoke of triangles. We thought that the therapeutic community could benefit from some suggestions for adopting a common language about triangles and for coming to a common understanding of them.

The usefulness of this book to you, we hope, will be threefold. First, it will benefit the whole psychotherapy community if it advances our ability both to see the ubiquity of triangles in emotional and relationship problems and to think and talk in terms of threes as well as in terms of individuals and dyads. Second, for those of you who already use the triangle concept in your practices, we hope it will sharpen and refine your understanding of triangles and give you some new ideas for using triangles as a way of intervening with the people you try to help. Third, for those of you who don't use the idea, we hope it will become a new weapon in your arsenal that will prove useful in many cases, but especially in those where you feel stuck. Thinking triangles can be very useful in getting unstuck in therapy and for moving off the dime with a case that's at an impasse.

We have organized the pages that follow into thirteen chapters, laced heavily with case material. The first chapter tells the story of how the notion of threesomes, triads, and eventually triangles came into family therapy and psychological thinking. Chapters 2 and 3 are our effort to explain and illustrate the importance for clinical work of thinking triangles. Chapters 4 through 6 explore triangles as *structure*, *process*, *movement*, and *function*.

In Chapters 7 through 12, we get into even more detail about clinical technique. Here we offer a typology of triangles most often seen in clinical practice with individuals (Chapters 7–8), couples (Chapters 9–10), and children and their families (Chapters 11–12), along with methods for intervention. We conclude in Chapter 13 with a summary of treatment methods.

The book is the product of more than a hundred years of the authors' combined clinical experience with families, couples, and individuals, of many hours spent refining the concepts of family systems theory and developing treatment protocols that evolve from the theory. Over the years, we've found the concept of the relationship triangle both the most challenging to refine as a concept and to translate into methods of clinical intervention. The pages that follow represent our best efforts. We don't believe they're the last word on triangles. We do believe they're a good beginning.

For the past twenty-two years, the Center for Family Learning in New Rochelle and then Rye Brook, New York, has been a place where family theory and treatment have flourished. The CFL environment has nurtured our ideas and our colleagues, friends, families, and patients have been our teachers. We're grateful to all these people for their contributions and understanding. We owe special thanks to the present faculty at the Center, especially to the members of the Marital Project—Nancy Edelman, Barbara Gewirtz, Donna Gundy, Wendy Michel, and Katherine Moseley—whose consultation on the clinical material used in this book was invaluable.

We are, of course, indebted to Murray Bowen, whose family systems theory and concepts blazed the trail on which we have traveled (though not always the same way that he did). It is with great respect and love that we remember him and the unique way he thought about people and their problems. We're especially grateful to Mike Nichols, our series editor at The Guilford Press. His generous contribution of time and his laser-beam criticism, tucked kindly into his wit, demanded our best efforts in return. His expertise in family systems and his wide knowledge of psychology allowed us to broaden the scope of our thinking. His love of writing and of good style always came through in his long letters of proposed changes. We're grateful as well to James McGee, professor of social work at the College of New Rochelle, who read our manuscript in its middle stages. His evaluation of the text's usefulness to students of clinical social work and to family therapists in training was particularly helpful. Finally, we thank our families, who have been patient, supportive, and nondemanding of our time as we worked on this project.

Contents

CHAPTER ONE

Relationship Triangles: Evolution of the Concept

At the very beginning—of your life, as soon as your conception became known, either your father, your mother, or both may have experienced you as an intruder. The fact of your existence may have overjoyed your father and presented a threat to your mother's career, making your father too eager for your arrival and your mother too anxious. Even before your conception, not-so-subtle pressure from your maternal grandmother may have led the campaign for your existence. At your birth, whatever genetic map was on your face was probably the stimulus for all kinds of loyalty-driven distinctions by well-meaning relatives. "He looks just like George's mother," says George's mother's sister.

From this perspective, we can see life not so much as a series of paths to be chosen, but as a maze of triangular shoals and reefs to be navigated around. As if this weren't difficult enough, you decided to become a psychotherapist—a professional sailing instructor. Every clinical presentation, every patient faces a mass of these triangular crosscurrents, and you're volunteering to help. Most systems psychotherapists have a mental file of their own experience of wrestling with relationship triangles. But whether you do a short-term solution or long-term growth model, the triangles are there, affecting your outcome.

Anna K. comes to mind. She was an 8-year-old waif of a girl with beautiful oversized brown eyes, destined to break a few hearts in the future. Her mother brought her to therapy at the suggestion of her third-grade teacher, who found her distracted, staring off into space, looking sad, and acting overtired at times in class. Anna was the youngest of three sisters. Her parents had divorced when she was 5. Since then, her mother had a new boyfriend, her father had moved from New York to California, and life went on.

At the first session, Anna asked her mother to stay in the room. She gave one-word answers but smiled with her eyes. Mrs. K. was motivated to get help, still felt guilty that she had "failed" in her mothering, and seemed caught between feelings of responsibility to her children, her job, and the demands of her new relationship. The therapist listened and asked questions, and at one point found himself wondering how Mr. K. could have left this very appealing 37-year-old woman and the little girl with the beautiful brown eyes. At the end of the session he suggested to Mrs. K. that perhaps the demands on her from her job and her new relationship had produced too much distance between her and her daughter. He proposed that perhaps some increase in relationship time with Anna, doing what Anna wanted to do, might improve their connection. If that happened, Anna might stop taking refuge in her daydreams and more actively and happily engage with her teacher and classmates. Or, at least the improved connection might result in Anna's sharing with her mother whatever was troubling her.

Upon their return for the follow-up appointment 3 weeks later, Mrs. K. reported that the situation was much worse. She had faithfully complied with the therapist's suggestions, but not only had Anna not improved at school, she had begun having temper tantrums at home. At this point, the therapist might have become defensively overresponsible and fallen into the trap of trying to fix something that he obviously didn't yet fully understand. Instead he listened to Mrs. K.'s story and asked about what she had tried and with what results. He asked if she had a theory about what had happened. She said she was at a loss to explain Anna's reaction and was discouraged and more worried than before.

The therapist turned to Anna and asked if her mother could leave for a while so that they could talk and draw some pictures. Anna agreed, and among the pictures she drew on the therapist's large new print pad was one of her family. She placed her father far to the left of the page; her mother and her mother's new boyfriend were together at the center; and her two older sisters were together closer to their father but down toward the bottom left-hand corner. Even more striking than the alignment of the people was the discrepancy in size between her oldest sister, Connie, and the rest of the people. The picture reminded the therapist of the line from Shakespeare's *Julius Caesar,* that she "doth bestride the narrow world like a colossus." He asked Anna about Connie. She wasn't very forthcoming; but she did say that Connie missed Daddy the most of anybody.

The therapist asked Anna to get her mother and then take some time to play with the toys in the waiting room while he and Mommy talked. Anna agreed and when she brought her mother in, the therapist asked her to show her mother her pictures. When Anna left the room, he used the family picture to devise a follow-up intervention. He suggested to Mrs. K. that the reason the first experiment had backfired was that it had increased the tension between Anna and her big sister, Connie, who was already of the opinion that Anna was spoiled rotten. He proposed that the information gathered from the first experiment, coupled with the information from Anna's family drawing, made it reasonable to devise a new test. In this one Mrs. K. would stop her increased attention to Anna and direct it instead toward her oldest daughter, Connie.

Mrs. K. complied with the therapist's advice and spent more time with Connie and less time with Anna. She was met with a significant dose of Connie's 13-year-old cynicism, and this occasioned her bringing Connie in for a few sessions. Now Connie and her mother had a chance to discuss how much Connie missed her father, was burdened by the child-care and other domestic responsibilities that her mother had given her, and felt criticized to boot. She told her mother that it especially hurt when Anna wouldn't cooperate and Mrs. K. wouldn't back her up. As if all that weren't enough, "who asked her to bring this new jerk into their lives?"

Mrs. K. and Connie did well with each other. Connie got more telephone time with her father and a spring vacation to visit him in California all by herself. Over the next 3 months, the tension between Anna and Connie decreased significantly. Anna's teacher reported great improvement, and Anna even began to help Connie with the housework.

A HISTORICAL PERSPECTIVE

A knowledge of triangles can sometimes produce amazing results, perhaps more times than you'd think. But then, we all know "triangles" works with kid problems. Freud knew this well before Bowen, Fogarty, Haley, and Minuchin reminded the rest of us. Freud cured Little Hans of his horse phobia by instructing his father on how the oedipal dilemma sets up a young boy to displace his fear of fatherly retaliation onto an animal.

> The boy had a phobia of horses, and as a result he refused to go out in the street. He expressed a fear that the horse would come into the room and bite him; and it turned out that this must be the punishment for a wish that the horse might fall down (that is, die). After the boy's fear of his father had been removed by reassurances, it became evident that he was struggling against wishes which had as their subject the idea of his father being absent (going away on a journey, dying). He regarded his father (as he made all too clear) as a competitor for the favors of his mother, towards whom the obscure foreshadowing of his budding sexual wishes were aimed. Thus he was situated in the typical attitude of a male child towards his parents to which we have given the name of the "Oedipus complex" and which we regard in general as the nuclear complex of the neuroses. The new fact we have learnt from the analysis of "Little Hans"—a fact with an important bearing upon totemism—is that in such circumstances children displace some of their feelings from their father on to an animal. . . . As soon as his anxiety began to diminish, he identified himself with the dreaded creature: he began to jump about like a horse and in his turn bit his father.[1]

The Philadelphia Child Guidance Clinic group of Salvador Minuchin, Jay Haley, Braulio Montalvo, Mariano Barragan, and others gave us the famous case they called "A Modern Little Hans."[2] Here an 8-year-old adopted boy was so afraid of dogs that his fear confined him to the house. Ironically the boy's father was a letter carrier, a job category whose conflictual relationship with dogs is legendary. The intervention strategy that Haley devised was so successful that it marked the clinical demonstration of the systemic aspects of children's symptoms.

The clinical pitfall of selling family therapy to families with a symptomatic child was dealt a damaging blow by the demonstration of structural techniques used for the presenting problem in this case.

---

[1] Freud (1913/1955, pp. 128–129).

[2] Haley (1987, pp. 244–261).

"A Modern Little Hans" beautifully shows the clinically induced structural alteration of a child-focused family using a strategy developed from the symptom. The result of the structural alteration was to alleviate the symptoms in the boy; the process shifted, and symptoms then emerged in his mother and in his parents' marital relationship. This shift automatically redefined the problem as a family problem rather than a child problem.

The Philadelphia group understood the central nuclear family triangle of the boy, his father, and his mother as follows: The relationship between the parents was distant but not openly conflictual. The relationship between mother and son was intense and overinvolved and that between father and son was extremely distant. The therapist's strategy combined two elements: (1) a prescription of the symptom with its paradoxical effects, and (2) the introduction of an object around which to organize the father–son relationship and overcome their distance from one another.

The actual therapeutic task called for the family to adopt a puppy, but it had to be a shy puppy, and the boy's job was to train the puppy to be friendly. His father, who as a mail carrier had all sorts of experience with dogs, was to help the boy train the puppy. Later, when they brought the puppy to the session, you could see the boy and his father playing with the puppy with obvious enjoyment during the therapy session. The unanticipated side effect was the observable developing depression in the boy's mother. The therapists had now defined this child's problem as a family problem.

Freud's case demonstrated the mechanism of displacement. The Philadelphia case showed not only displacement but also the absorption by a child of parental anxiety and marital tension. The latter had been proposed earlier by Murray Bowen in his work with schizophrenia when he postulated the existence of a *multigenerational projection process*.[3]

In his pioneering work on schizophrenia at the Menninger Clinic, Bowen paid attention to the intense, symbiotic attachment between mothers and their schizophrenic children. Besides their intense dependence on one another, he observed a striking pattern of behavior. This pattern consisted of cycles of intense closeness followed by extreme distance. These cycles occurred quite predictably over time. Bowen thought that the cycles of closeness and distance

---

[3] Kerr (1988, Chap. 8).

were driven by corresponding internal states of separation anxiety and fear of being taken over, or incorporation anxiety.

Later we will see how profoundly important, and often misunderstood, these cycles of closeness and distance are. Their roots in psychoanalytic theory led some family therapists to misunderstand Bowen's efforts to build a systems theory. The link between these cycles of closeness and distance and triangles becomes clear when you ask to whom (or to what) people go when they distance from someone with whom they have been close.

Vicki P. was a financial analyst for a large mutual funds company. She was 37 when she came to our clinic at the suggestion of Debbie, her closest friend. Debbie had successfully turned her life and her marriage around 2 years earlier and gave her therapist a big share of the credit for her success. Vicki said she wanted "some of whatever it was that Debbie had gotten."

When Vicki and Bob first met, Bob was the first to feel the chemistry. He pursued Vicki, and as their courtship went on, both of them felt cradled in the warmth of their mutual attraction. Since each of them was more than five hundred miles away from their families of origin, they enjoyed the romantic cocoon without interference. A year into the courtship, with both being over 30, they decided to get married and traveled to Vicki's parents' home in Michigan to announce their engagement. During her childhood, adolescence, and early adulthood, Vicki had been very close (some might say too close) to her father, Don. In fact she had moved to New York to put some physical distance into their relationship. The maneuver worked because Vicki felt much less controlled and pressured by him.

Vicki had met Bob 2 years after moving to New York. During the planning for the wedding, Bob felt a little intimidated by his future father-in-law, but he chalked it up to "one of those family things" and left Vicki with the responsibility of dealing with it. Having put off their marriage until their 30s, these two highly successful professionals had saved enough money to buy a home right away. Both of them shared an interest in architecture and loved older homes. Don had fostered this interest in his daughter and was himself a jack-of-all-trades when he wasn't running his own electrical supply house. When Vicki and Bob moved into their house, Don offered to come to New York and help them with the beginning of their renovations. He arrived on a Friday night, and the three of them had a lovely dinner together. By the time Saturday mid-morning came, Vicki noticed that Bob's interest in the project was waning quickly. His lack of participation worsened as the weekend progressed, and culminated in an emotional outburst from Bob that resulted in a fight with his father-in-law. Don returned to Michigan feeling that Bob did not respect him. Whenever Vicki would urge Bob to apologize to her father, he would say, "You manage your own family, okay? He's your father; I don't have to love him."

Vicki managed the growing tension in the marriage by devoting more and more of her time to her work and her son. The couple would have occasional warm and pleasant Sundays with their son, but they never came close to melting the new ice in their relationship. Bob became more invested in his job and spent less and less time at home. Finally, Vicki became alarmed at their distance from one another, and she took her friend Debbie into her confidence. When Vicki approached Bob about going to a therapist, he informed her he wasn't sure he still loved her and wasn't certain their relationship had a future. Vicki's strategy for dealing with this was to continue to urge Bob to come to therapy, but she was feeling hopeless about it helping. She moved toward the solution that had worked with her father and openly talked about the possibility of a split-cities marriage—a geographic cure.

Initially Bob responded with indifference; he viewed her idea as just another in a long line of empty threats. Yet when he read the letter confirming Vicki's appointment for an interview in Washington, he panicked and begged her to reconsider. He promised to come to therapy to try to heal the rift. Vicki made the initial call to the clinic and came alone at first for two reasons. She wasn't sure if she had enough emotional resilience left to go around the track one more time. Besides, she was afraid that joining Bob in a therapist's office would be a signal to him that, having made another token gesture, he could return to his perpetually distant ways The therapist encouraged Vicki to stay on track, to go through with her interview in Washington, but to remain open to sustained, concrete effort on Bob's part.

We can easily track the alternating cycles of closeness and distance between Vicki and Bob, from their initial meeting at a cocktail party, to the threatened end of their marriage 8 years later. The triangles present include the explicit triangles of Vicki, her father, and Bob, and Vicki, her son, and Bob. In the background (the extended family closet, you might say) loomed Bob's conflictual relationship with his parents and brothers that he had handled with distance and emotional cutoff. These silent triangles in Bob's family were every bit as much a part of the clinical picture as the active and obvious ones in Vicki's family. The therapist must be aware of this symmetry of dysfunction in order to engage both parties in the work of therapy in a way that doesn't blame one or the other or indict one's family of origin over the other's.

Right now Vicki and Bob are living 300 miles away from each other, their son is with Vicki, and they spend alternating weekends together in the two cities. Progress in therapy has been modest, with the major obstacle being the triangles with Vicki's father and their son.

If you watch for the same cycles of closeness and distance in your own life, with parents, spouses, children, good friends, and work associates, you'll find them. They are just less intense and less extreme than Murray Bowen's mother–child pairs, or even Vicki and Bob. Some are obvious and their reasons clear; some seem to happen for no reason at all. The friend you couldn't wait to talk to about something that happened last week is mildly irritating today when he interrupts your work to chat. The baby whose demands yesterday made you think you would go crazy, you now are delighted to play with. The lover you couldn't keep your hands off last night is a real turnoff this morning, for some reason not entirely clear. A little boy eagerly seeks out his mother when he thinks she is trying to avoid him or when she seems relieved that Grampa has come to take him out for the afternoon. Later the boy seems less needy of her time, more indifferent to her, until in adolescence he becomes positively arrogant about how she needed him more than he needed her. He becomes resistant to her requests to do things together, and his friends are a lot more important to spend time with. The importance of these kinds of observations is the way they reveal the instability of dyads. *It is the instability of dyads that produces relationship triangles.*

Tom Fogarty took Bowen's observations on cycles of closeness and distance and, rather than focusing on the internal need to be connected or anxiety about being engulfed, he focused on the relationship movement by each individual. People have three movement options in a relationship: They can move toward the other person, they can move away, or they can stand still. This movement is not theoretical—it can be observed by the participants and by the therapist. The movement is driven by an increase in the level of emotional arousal of the individuals and by their emotional response (their emotional reactivity) to the behavior of the other person or to their perception of the other person's emotional state. Emotional arousal in the individual, together with the reactive movement it drives, is the fuel that feeds the activation of triangles. *Emotional reactivity* is the key to seeing how unstable dyads produce triangles.

The day he learned that his superiors had passed him over for promotion at the post office, Fred S. felt as if someone had driven a spike through his dream of self-respect. He couldn't wait for the workday to end so he could get out of that alien place and go home to seek solace in his world-class stamp collection. He was delighted to find that his wife Gerry and son Sean weren't home yet, and he headed directly for his den. Gerry and Sean got in 3 hours later, and Gerry knew Fred was home because his jacket was hanging in the hall closet. She also sensed something was wrong, and she went off to find him. Sean, a gangly and shy 14-year-old, used the opportunity to make a beeline for his room and his beloved stereo.

The relationship of each of these three is easy to follow. Each of them was moving in a way that served the purpose of calming their emotional state and making the environment as emotionally safe as possible. They had not yet activated the potential triangle. Gerry was moving toward Fred. When she arrived at his den, she found he had locked the door. Her emotional arousal continued to escalate. "Fred, are you in there?" "Yes, I'm fine," Fred replied without unlocking the door. After a few more questions followed by one-word answers, Gerry moved away toward the kitchen to get dinner. She put some leftover baked ziti and garlic bread from their favorite Italian restaurant in the microwave. She still felt annoyed over Fred's nonresponse to her, decided she wasn't going to let him get to her, heaved a sigh and went to Sean's room to help him with his homework.

When his mother entered his room, Sean left complaining that he was hungry. Mary then lost her cool and began to yell about his homework and insisted on knowing what his assignments were. Since Fred can't stand loud noises, he emerged from his retreat, sized up the situation, and joined Gerry in castigating Sean. The movement patterns are clear; They have activated the triangle, and we can trace the activation back to emotional reactivity.

In his schizophrenia project at the National Institute of Mental Health, Bowen documented the crucial role of the distant, uninvolved father in the families of schizophrenics. Fathers, he noticed, were intensely reactive to mothers' anxiety and behaved reactively when they sensed an increase in their wives' upset. They might join with their wives in worry about or criticism of their schizophrenic children; they might distance even farther to escape the increased tension; what they never did was move toward their schizophrenic children. It was this phenomenon that Bowen was talking about when he first used the term *triad,* and later *triangle.*

I began work on this basic concept in 1955. By 1956 the research group was thinking and talking about "triads." As the concept evolved, it came to include much more than the meaning of the conventional term *triad,* and we therefore had a problem communicating with those who assumed they knew the meaning of triad. I chose *triangle* in order to convey that this concept has specific meaning beyond that implied in triad.[4]

From these clinical observations, Bowen was attempting to go beyond Freud's thinking about triangles. Bowen's view was that triangles weren't limited to oedipal developments; they were more generic than that. In fact, whenever tension exists in a dyad, emotional forces begin to operate in a way that brings about a stabilizing relationship triangle. For example, Bowen observed that the tension existing between the schizophrenic child and his or her mother was picked up on by the father as upset in the mother. This in turn raised the father's level of anxiety, which moved him to try to put a lid on his wife's upset—going to any extreme to placate her, including denying her part in her conflict with her child. The child would thus feel abandoned by both parents, shut out, criticized, and locked into the position of the one with a problem.

Davy N. spent a lot of time with his mother, even for a 5-year-old. Mrs. N. was especially involved with him about his school work. Davy had a serious learning disability, and in spite of specialized tutoring with professionals, Mrs. N. was concerned that he needed her help, too. Mr. N. vehemently disagreed. He thought his wife was making Davy into a "momma's boy." Mr. and Mrs. N. didn't allow themselves to get into their differences about Davy (or, for that matter, about anything else). Mrs. N. focused her energies on her son's problems, while Mr. N. stayed distant from both of them, concentrating on work and his train collection.

Bowen began to see that clinical problems were invariably embedded in these three-person structures (e.g., the schizophrenic young adult and both parents). Unlike Freud, however, Bowen rejected the idea that the energy driving the emotional process in these structures was always libidinal. Bowen postulated that the driving force in triangles was an anxious attachment carried to the extreme. He called this anxious attachment *fusion*: a symbiotic attachment and blurring of boundaries between two people in which the transmission

---

[4] Bowen (1978, p. 373).

of anxiety is so intense that both people become convinced that they can't survive without the other. Such symbiotic attachment, or fusion, is manifested behaviorally in cycles of closeness and distance between mother and schizophrenic offspring; they move toward and away from each other in what looks like a never-ending search for a comfortable relationship space. They act like a set of magnets that attract one another if they are at a certain distance but that begin to repel one another the second they get too close.

These same cycles of closeness and distance appear, although perhaps in less extreme form, in all dyadic relationships—parent and child, brother and sister, husband and wife, even friend and friend. These behavioral cycles are reactions to internal anxiety: separation anxiety compelling attempts at closeness, incorporation anxiety driving distance. This dynamic is the key to the inherent *instability* of the relationship dyad.

In therapy, Bowen worked with triangles in two ways. One approach was to place himself as therapist in the position of a potentially triangled third party. Then he would work at staying detriangled while remaining connected to each person in the dyad.[5] Indeed, he maintained that this is the essence of marital therapy: Stay connected with both spouses, but don't let them triangle you. In practice, Bowen would connect with each person, one at a time, often choosing to begin with the overfunctioning or more motivated partner. He would ask nonconfrontational questions, verify facts, and hear feelings. He would form each question to stimulate cognition rather than squeeze for feeling. His objective was to develop and hear out through questions and answers the perceptions and opinions of each partner, without siding emotionally with either one. It's taking sides that keeps triangles going.

Staying out of triangles sounds simple, but it can't be accomplished just by stating "I'm not going to take sides with either one of you," or "I'm not going to get into a triangle with you two." Emotional neutrality *can* be a trap if the therapist walks on eggs so as not to give the appearance of being stymied by the partners' conflict. In fact, anxiety about remaining neutral paradoxically *catches* therapists in a triangular trap because they lose the ability to move freely between the partners and are paralyzed. The therapist's ability to remain emotionally calm in the face of intense feelings is critical to avoiding both

---

[5] Kerr and Bowen (1988, p. 145).

the trap of taking sides and the trap of neutrality paralysis. Therapists' awareness of their personal triggers can help, as can extensive experience at dealing with invitations to get into triangles in their clinical work and in their personal lives.

Bowen's second approach to resolving triangles was to work with the best-functioning individual in a system. He would coach that person to detriangle him- or herself—that is, to act on her own beliefs and values without cutting off from the other people in the system. Bowen's now-famous paper on his own efforts to differentiate in his family of origin showed how to do this.[6] Remember, without becoming paranoid, that every individual or couple you deal with is a problem in search of a triangle. Patients' efforts to solve their problems with triangles can be very challenging when a therapist is working with individual patients and coaching them to function better and be better connected in their personal and occupational relationship systems. A therapist trained to think about triangles remains vigilant to the number and intensity of the triangles that are in the room. This is true even with individual patients, and it includes the potential triangles that involve the therapist.

The idea of triangles began with work on schizophrenia, but its widespread acceptance and use in family therapy came about in work on child-centered families at the Philadelphia Child Guidance Clinic. There the idea became less process oriented and more structural in focus. Therapists saw triangles as the direct result of a blurring of boundaries between family subsystems rather than as the result of emotional process and reactivity. They thought that the shape of triangles was fixed rather than constantly in motion. They thought that a triangle operated as a single modular unit over two generations rather than being connected with a whole series of interlocking triangles, some of which might involve one or three generations.

Thomas Fogarty, influenced by Bowen but less enamored of psychoanalytic thinking, was the first to focus on relationship movement in the study of triangles. He described how individuals move toward and away from each other in response to their discomfort about being too close or too distant. He pointed out that movement created the structure of a triangle: An individual moves toward a third person as he or she moves away from the second member of a dyad (for example, a husband moves toward an affair as he moves

---

[6] Bowen (1978, p. 529 ff).

away from his wife). In other words, Fogarty viewed triangles as a short-circuiting mechanism that serves the purposes of avoiding discomfort with intimacy and of avoiding discomfort with facing conflictual issues.

Fogarty noticed that couples with young children who came to him about their marriages commonly shared a similar dynamic that underlay the variations in their stories. When these couples were first married, there had been enough love and affection to satisfy both of them. When the family expanded with the birth of a baby, they had less time, less energy, less privacy, and less freedom. Mothering consumed the wife, and she became less wife and more mother. As the husband moved toward her and tried to restore the original state of affairs, he failed. The twosome had become a threesome (and, at least potentially, a triangle). These husbands generally understood that the *status quo ante* was gone forever—but, they still missed their wives. Often they dealt with their loss by getting more absorbed in work and career, becoming more distant from both mother and child. Now the triangle had become a problem as it became an integral part of the way the family was operating. Detriangling here meant getting the father to move toward his child and step up his fathering.

Fogarty's observations of patients in his office led him to think that certain individuals may have greater tendencies toward separation anxiety *or* incorporation anxiety. This produces behavior that he labeled "emotional pursuit" or "emotional distance."[7] The partners of emotional pursuers perceive them as threatening incorporation, which activates the distancers' anxiety and intensifies their distancing behavior. The partners of emotional distancers perceive them as threatening abandonment (separation), triggering the pursuers' anxiety and intensifying their pursuit. The more intense the anxiety on either part, the more likely are efforts to stabilize the dyad by activation of a triangle.

Fogarty's primary method of intervention was to change the direction of people's movement in triangles and thus change the triangle's structure. Changing the structure by changing the movement would give people a different way of operating in their families. It would also uncover the issues people are avoiding through the triangle and allow them to deal with those issues in therapy. For example, if a mother habitually directed the details of her child's life as her husband distanced from both of them, Fogarty would prescribe

---

[7] Fogarty (1979).

mother's pulling back from the child and father's moving in toward the child for caretaking or relationship time. If both parents made good faith efforts to comply with the prescription, they would reverse the flow of their movement. As they did that, Fogarty would coach them to monitor their internal emotional reactions to that changing movement. Their old movement, he thought, was a way of dissipating emotional discomfort. This new movement would go counter to the inclinations of their emotional states. It would also go counter to what their own experience has taught them will give them relief from their uncomfortable internal states. At this point, people start to get in touch with these uncomfortable internal states and are likely to experience more anxiety or depression. If the family has complied with the restructuring prescription, there will be a structural alteration in the triangle with a resulting relief of the presenting symptom. When relief of the presenting symptom happens, a new set of symptoms can appear, whose existence the presenting symptom had been camouflaging. The new set of symptoms might include underground marital conflict, a husband's depression, or a wife's alcoholism.

Salvador Minuchin and Jay Haley, working with Mariano Barragan, Braulio Montalvo, and others, developed structural and strategic methods for dealing with triangles. Their major method of intervention was to use the symptoms and promote a structural shift to relieve the symptom bearer of his plight.

Minuchin thought about the structure of the family as a whole, including the common finding that mothers are enmeshed with their children, whereas fathers are disengaged. Thus any attempt to deal with Johnnie's misbehavior without dealing with the fact that his mother isn't strict with him would be unlikely to succeed. But failing to see mother's lack of strictness as a part of her overinvolvement with her son, and to see that his is related to her underinvolvement with her husband—and his with her—would also be likely to fail. This principle is illustrated in Minuchin's case of Sally Brown, a 10-year-old hospitalized with anorexia nervosa.[8] Minuchin created a family crisis in the session around Sally's eating—a crisis that revealed the overprotectiveness of Sally's parents, their lack of involvement with each other, father's peripheral role in the family, and mother's intense involvement with the child subsystem. Insisting that the parents allow Sally, with the guidance of her pediatrician, to

---

[8] Minuchin (1974).

make her own choices of the food she wanted to eat relieved Sally's anorexia and was the first move in restructuring the family. The restructuring required transforming both the spousal subsystem and the sibling subsystem by establishing appropriate boundaries between them and effective communication within and between them.

By contrast, Haley focused more narrowly on what he called cross-generational coalitions. He developed a three-step strategy to deal with them.

1. Hook up the disengaged parent with the dependent child, in order to separate the enmeshed parent and child.
2. Move the parents closer together.
3. Challenge the symptom directly, usually with some sort of paradoxical prescription.

For example, in the case of the boy with the dog phobia, we saw the boy locked in a triangle that had mother and son overly close and father in a distant position. The therapists devised a treatment strategy, getting the father to teach the son how to deal with dogs. Thus they used the symptom strategically to create an affiliation between father and son, closing off the distance and changing the structure of the triangle.

Minuchin's and Haley's structural and strategic approaches to triangles came to dominate family therapy. As the focus became more strategic and less structural, Haley moved away from triangles. He began to work on strategies for individuals, as pioneered by Milton Erickson.

The next stage in the development of the triangle concept came from Philip Guerin's connection with Murray Bowen. Guerin's first contact with Bowen occurred during the second year of his psychiatric residency at Georgetown. This was in 1967, 8 years after Bowen left the National Institute of Mental Health to come to Georgetown. After hearing Bowen's lecture on schizophrenia and the family, Guerin sought supervision on a case of a 19-year-old schizophrenic woman and her family. Guerin had been carrying this case at D.C. General Hospital since the early weeks of his first year of residency. He thought that his patient was caught in an extremely ambivalent relationship with her mother. The mother appeared cold toward her daughter and burdened by her. The father, a career public health officer, was anxious and seemed to have no opinion about his daughter or his wife or the relationship they had with one another. He seemed afraid of losing his wife and of having life pass his daughter by.

Guerin brought this triangle to Bowen and asked his help in fixing it, with the hope that this young woman could somehow be freed to live a more normal life. Bowen suggested treating this family with network therapy. At that time Ross Speck and Carolyn Attneave[9] were developing a method of "de-escalating" schizophrenics and their families by having them form social networks that would meet regularly with their therapist. Bowen was trying out this idea mainly because he saw it as potentially defusing the intensity of the symbiotic attachment between mothers and their schizophrenic children—almost as if the network relationships could create a series of interlocking triangle circuits that could drain off some tension in the family's central triangle. Guerin saw the idea as offering an artificially formed extended family.

Bowen's supervision was at once vague and pregnant with wisdom, but it lacked a step-by-step explication of the concept of triangles and how to use them clinically. It was at this time that Guerin became committed to taking some of these new family systems ideas and elaborating them in ways that made them more understandable and more usable in day-to-day clinical practice. Bowen's ideas about triangles made Guerin aware of several professional and personal triangles at a developmentally critical time for him. As a medical student he had formed a close attachment to the chairman of the Department of Psychiatry at Georgetown, Richard Steinbach. Steinbach was an imposing paragon with a deep, resonant voice and conservative analytic beliefs formed in his native Georgia and at the Baltimore Psychoanalytic Institute. He was a strong influence on Guerin's choice of psychiatry as a specialization. Even though Bowen was an important member of the Georgetown faculty, the unorthodoxy of his ideas and their influence on young residents like Guerin troubled Steinbach. In addition, Guerin was in analytic therapy (but not psychoanalysis) twice a week dealing with his idealization of important internalized objects. The notion of triangles broadened his perspective to include an appreciation of how he was caught in triangles with these objects (like the one with Bowen and Steinbach). All these converging forces formed the beginnings of Guerin's ideas about triangles being a by-product of the struggle about "primacy of attachment and hierarchy of influence."

---

[9] Speck and Attneave (1973).

Guerin took the combined triangles of his nuclear and extended families and his professional life to Bowen for relationship coaching. Thus he fled the couch, and eventually Washington, as well, to take refuge in the wonderful chaos of a residency at the Albert Einstein College of Medicine in the Bronx. During his last year of residency at Georgetown, Guerin had gotten together with Tom Fogarty and became interested in his ideas about movement, pursuit, and distance in relationships—ideas that Fogarty presented at the Georgetown Family Symposium. Guerin saw these as operational concepts for Bowen's ideas about cycles of closeness and distance. He was particularly interested in Fogarty's application of these ideas to experiments aimed at altering the structure of relationship triangles, especially child-centered triangles.

When Guerin arrived at Einstein, he contacted Fogarty and, with the permission of the administration, invited him to collaborate in the development of family systems ideas. Guerin brought a relationship process orientation from his work with Bowen to join with Fogarty's notion of the importance of tracking movement in the structure of relationship triangles.

In the late 1970s and early 1980s, Fogarty's midlife frustration with the recycling of symptoms in emotional pursuers, and his own philosopher core, took him into the clinical study of the existential experience of inner emptiness. Fogarty viewed this as an emotional state caused by the realization of the limitations in what individuals could expect to get from their relationships.

At this point Fogarty's dysthymia and Guerin's cyclothymia took them in different directions. Guerin thought Bowen and Fogarty were going off on the tangents of societal regression (Bowen) and individual emptiness (Fogarty). He turned his own efforts, along with his colleagues Leo Fay, Susan Burden, and Judith Kautto, to emphasizing the centrality of relationship triangles in systems psychotherapy. This emphasis appeared first in work on child- and adolescent-centered families,[10] and then on the marital relationship.[11] They elaborated on the mechanisms of triangle activation and combined a structural and process orientation. They introduced the ideas of hierarchy of influence and primacy of attachment and showed the clinical usefulness of a symptom-based typology of triangles.

---

[10] Guerin and Gordon (1984).

[11] Guerin, Fay, Burden, and Kautto (1987).

In their marital model, Guerin and his colleagues developed methods of intervention for dealing with relationship triangles. The techniques proposed by this group include:

1. Identifying the key triangle and surfacing the emotional process in it by the introduction of relationship experiments, either through directly prescribed structural alterations, or indirectly by asking process questions (e.g., "What would happen if you turned over your son to your husband?");
2. Coaching each person in the triangle (or a single individual when therapy doesn't have access to the rest of the triangle) to change his or her part, also by relationship experiments;
3. Reinforcing progress by addressing the major interlocking triangles (for example, untangling an extramarital affair triangle can reveal an active, but up to now submerged, in-law triangle that must also be addressed).

The methods of treating emotional dysfunction through triangles developed by Minuchin, Haley, and the other structural and strategic therapists, focused on structural alterations with the goal of symptom relief. The methods developed and used by Bowen, Fogarty, and Guerin include structural alterations for symptom relief and a focus on bringing to the surface the emotional process that occurs within triangles. The latter approach has a major advantage: It gives therapeutic access to the underlying individual and dyadic processes that have been driving the presenting symptom. Unless the underlying processes are opened up and dealt with, symptom relief turns out to be just that: temporary improvement with frustrating cycles of recurrence. The symptoms in the child in the family, for example, may be relieved. Yet only by dealing with the triangle will the marital conflict, father's dependence on mother and his fear of rejection, and mother's fear of abandonment be revealed.

Changes in the health care delivery system predicated on the demands of managed care are now demanding a form of clinical practice that focuses almost exclusively on symptom relief. Like most changes, this has both its upside and its downside. On the upside, psychiatry and psychotherapy in particular have needed for a long time to pay more attention to the management and relief of symptoms. Managed care will force practitioners to remove the flab from psychotherapy. Expanding the observing ego and producing healthier relationship systems are desirable goals, but they'll have to be achieved by

more efficient methods. On the downside, there are many clinical situations in which medication and brief cognitive and behavioral management aren't going to be sufficient to the task. Just prescribing
Prozac or giving some advice simply isn't going to be effective for everybody.

Clinicians are already faced with the dilemma of choosing between methods of containment and methods that move to uncover
underlying emotional process. And there have always been therapists
who prefer brief to protracted therapy. Short doesn't have to mean
naive, however. The useful thing about triangles is that they are an essential ingredient in your conceptual understanding of the problem
and in your clinical intervention whether you're doing short-term
therapy and symptom management or you're doing longer-term individual or relationship work.

CHAPTER TWO

The Relevance of Triangles in Clinical Context

Life has treated every psychotherapist at one time or another to the observation that all mental health professionals are in the business because of their personal problems. This caricature has some truth to it. Many of us became interested in this field through perhaps an experience with a personal bout of depression, a childhood burdened by prolonged enuresis, an adolescence troubled by nonacceptance, a parent or grandparent or clergyman with a drinking problem. Still, it's also true that the complex nuances of personality—the self-centeredness of some, the intrusiveness of others—have tugged at our curiosity or troubled our souls. We came to love playing with the idea that the compulsive aspects of personality in ourselves or others may be linked to struggles during psychosexual development.

Our teachers have trained us to think, when dealing clinically with depression, about early childhood loss or deprivation repeated in later life. We think about repressed anger in middle age, or loss of status and function while struggling with the inevitability of old age. It is a simple enough step to move from thinking about the biological predisposition and psychological trauma of individuals to the tension and conflict in their relationships. Parents with a conflictual marriage and battles with siblings are easy to see as relevant. However, even with obvious triangles like extramarital affairs or bossy mothers-in-law, it is easier to think about twos rather than threes: Joe Blow and his mother-in-law; Suzy Q. and her latest lover. We tend to think about ones and twos—individuals and dyads—and this in spite of the fact that from the moment of conception we and everyone else are smack in the middle of the most important triangle of our lives.

We need to be trained to think about threes—triangles—as well as about individuals and dyads and to move freely in therapy from one level to the other. Mommy tells the 2-year-old, "No-no," and she quickly shifts her gaze to Daddy probing for a crack in the wall of parental authority. The 16-year-old whose father told him he can't have the car for a Saturday afternoon drive goes to the other side of the house to ask his mother if she needs anything at the store. "If I can't get it from Dad, there's always Mom," he thinks. The *instinct* to triangle is always there, but our *thinking* remains linear or dyadic.

Therapists like to think of themselves as knowledgeable, understanding, and supportive beings. These are all desirable characteristics, but remember that every individual who walks into our office, whether advantaged, attractive, and articulate, or traumatized, downtrodden, and disheveled, is to some extent looking for validation of his or her victimhood. Validation of feelings aroused by stressful or traumatic experiences is essential to good psychotherapy, but helping patients to objectify their experiences, modify their distortions, and accept responsibility for their own part in their problems and in the resolution of those problems is just as critical. A working knowledge of triangles is essential to this therapeutic balancing act. Just keep in mind that no matter how psychologically minded and apparently self-focused a couple in marital conflict may appear, more than likely one or both of them are looking to transfer their competition at home, at the office, or on the tennis court to a get-the-therapist-on-my-side contest.

The work of Minuchin and others has given family therapy wide credibility by demonstrating clinically and on videotape the effectiveness of treating a child's symptom as a part of the family system. Minuchin's success in alerting us to the importance of the subsystems and boundaries that structure family life made most therapists aware that a child who misbehaves or gets depressed is probably caught up in an unhealthy triangle with her or his parents. In practice, however, we often blur this kind of insight, and therapists fall back on thinking that the "real" problem is between the parents. After all, we've been programmed to think parents are responsible for their children's well-being; anyway, if there weren't tension in the marriage before symptom development in the child, there certainly would be afterwards. Furthermore, the traditional child guidance model viewed parents either as the source of the problem or as the potential undoers of therapeutic progress. In the early days of family therapy, in an attempt to broaden the context of the child's symptoms, the tension in the parental relationship, which may or may not have existed before the child's symptoms, was a too-easy explanation for the clinical difficulty. All these factors, perhaps coupled with our own ambivalence toward our own parents, may make this an irresistible trap for a therapist.

Instead of keeping the triangle (all three people) in mind, therapists just shift away from the child to the marriage. It's a lot easier to think about individuals and dyads, victims and villains, than it is to keep in mind the complexity of all three people and their mutual influence.

THREE TYPES OF TRIANGLES

Clinicians of all stripes and persuasions have found it easiest to see triangles as a relevant way to understand cases that present with a problem in a child or adolescent. The next easiest kind of case for most clinicians to see the relevance of triangles is marital cases, especially those involving affairs and with in-law problems. Often the most difficult places to see triangles, however, are individual cases.

Child- or Adolescent-Centered Triangles

In child and adolescent cases, clinicians have seen triangles as an indication of a need for restructuring techniques, and many of those techniques have been strategic in nature. Such restructuring has often given rapid symptom relief in child- and adolescent-centered families, and so it has been a valuable tool in the armamentarium of family therapy. What restructuring leaves behind, however, is the clinical awareness of the emotional *process* that goes on within the structure of the triangle. Unless that process is dealt with along with the restructuring, the unresolved triangle lies dormant even after symptom relief, ready to be reactivated.

Haley and Barragan's case of the boy with the dog phobia, with which we began, illustrates this point very well. The symptom (the boy's reluctance to leave the house) gets resolved because of a brilliant strategic move to restructure the primary parental triangle. But as mother loosens her attachment to her son, the appearance of a sadness and mild depression begins to manifest itself in her. This turn of events represents externalization of an underlying conflict in the marriage and an internal upset in the mother, both of which drive the triangle involving the boy. It is important for the therapist to pay attention to the relationship process that structural interventions unearth. Otherwise the therapist will miss the latent relationship and individual conditions that may be driving the triangle.

Marital Triangles

Guerin, Fay, Burden, and Kautto reported on their clinical experience with marital conflict in 1987. *The evaluation and treatment of marital conflict* is about the theory and treatment of marital dysfunction and was the result of many years of wrestling with the difficult work of sitting with bitter couples and trying to help them. These therapists found that, in marriages with a modest degree of conflict of short duration and relatively low intensity, work on the dyad itself is usually sufficient to produce good results. However, in cases of severe marital conflict, with long duration and high intensity, the therapist almost always must locate, define, and resolve the triangles surrounding the marital relationship. Otherwise, in the highest percentage of cases, treatment either fails or produces only short-term improvement with rapid recycling and, perhaps ultimately, disintegration. In fact, it was this discovery about triangles in treating severely disrupted couples that motivated us to look at triangles themselves as a unique and distinct entity.

Work on triangles in marital therapy makes sense to many clinicians, especially in cases where extramarital affairs or interfering in-laws are the presenting problem. Often, however, marital triangles aren't as easy to see or to work with in treatment as child-centered triangles are. Therapists find themselves bogged down in the morass of dyadic wars. They are unable to see or do anything about the triangles that are reinforcing the wars and making a negotiated settlement difficult. People do displace unresolved conflict. Husbands and wives can (and do) displace unresolved conflicts from their own families into the marriage. (Take the example of the wife who is convinced, with compelling evidence, that her parents and siblings don't love her and never have. She gives up on them and then fights the battle of "You don't really care about me" with her husband.) Similarly, a spouse can displace anger, resentment, and bitterness toward the other spouse onto a child, making that child the issue between them. ("If she would just be stricter with our son instead of excusing everything he does," for example. Or, "If he would be more understanding of our daughter.") The marital treatment is going to fail unless those unresolved issues are dealt with in the relationships where they belong.

Individual Dysfunction and Triangles

When we are dealing in therapy with individuals who have been refractory to other modalities of treatment, good results can follow if we understand the refractoriness as the result of patients being caught in one or more triangles. When individuals are caught in triangles, their freedom of movement is severely circumscribed. We have found that working on detriangling individuals has powerful consequences for producing significant improvement in the presenting problem and in resolving underlying issues. Such detriangling can be done either by coaching or by bringing one or more of the other members of the triangle into the treatment room. The challenge for the therapist is to keep thinking about triangles. It is hard enough in child-centered and marital cases, but it is especially difficult in individual cases.

In some situations, families and therapists perceive the symptom as almost 100% in the individual. Such situations occur when one person is hospitalized, or if the symptom is as dramatic as a suicide attempt, or if the person stays home from work, or doesn't bathe or get dressed. Triangles are present, but they may be hidden or obscured by the severity of the symptom in one person. In these situations, all one can do is treat the individual symptom and keep in mind that there are underlying dyadic and triangular structures and processes. As the individual symptom abates, these structures and processes will become more apparent—if you know where to look for them.

For example, Pamela B., a 39-year-old attorney, was hospitalized for cocaine and alcohol addiction. Pamela had been "partying" on weekends with her husband, Jerome, and friends for 2 years before she began using cocaine during the week. Not using during the week had been a rule she and Jerome had made to keep things "recreational." But Pamela was under growing pressure from a burgeoning law practice, she was anxious to make partner, and she thought Jerome was more elusive and irritated with her than ever. The calm she got from a quick snort early in the morning, before a meeting, or late at night when Jerome was asleep and not interested in sex, was magnetic and therefore relaxing.

One day she became hysterical at the office when her secretary was late typing an important contract. Her outburst was so intense that a frightened coworker called 911. Pamela ended up in the emergency room of a large teaching hospital that happened to have a 28-day detoxification and rehabilitation program. It was only in the ER that Pamela realized how much she had gotten out of control. During her first few days in the hospital, Pamela went through the nightmare of detox. When she wasn't vomiting, she writhed in pain from stomach cramps. Finally, on the 4th day, barely able to move, she began the slow and difficult work of accepting that she was an addict and that her life had become unmanageable.

From childhood on, Pamela had found ways of alleviating emotional pain and discomfort. Her father had left the family when she was 5, and her mother had begun heavy drinking. Pamela daydreamed her way through those years. When she was a young teen, her mother married a man who was much younger and very demanding. Then Pamela went out as much as she could to smoke pot and drink with friends. She discovered sex when she realized that guys found her very pretty. With a wry smile she claimed that she was the original "sex, drugs, and rock-and-roll" girl. Pamela left home at 18 and came to New York to begin a modeling career. Before long she met Jerome. Their first date lasted 5 days, ending in a "coked-out stupor" in Jerome's cabin in the Adirondacks.

During the second stage of her treatment, as her head began to clear, Pamela saw that her cocaine addiction was tied up with a severe marital problem of many years' duration. Pamela had never asserted herself with Jerome, to let him know when something bothered or angered her. Instead, she frequently disappeared from home and would call to tell him she was on her way but never arrive. She was spending her time in the arms of another lover—cocaine. Her pattern of distancing and self-destructive behavior was an old one that went back to her inability to confront or talk directly to her mother, father, sister, or brother. *They* had all talked with one another about their concerns with Pamela. *She* had kept all her anger to herself. She had never dealt with any of them honestly and straightforwardly; instead, she would head for the hills, using drugs and alcohol as her transportation. The relationship triangles didn't cause Pamela's addictions or acting out, but the structure and processes of the triangles within her marriage and family of origin helped perpetuate the pattern.

There are many ways in which the idea of relationship triangles is clinically useful. For one, thinking about a case in terms of the triangles in it gives the therapist a road map for early intervention. If, for example, a therapist sees a mother excessively close to a child, with the father distant, the therapist knows that one of the first things that requires clinical attention may be to cut down the over closeness and reduce the distance. Explaining the triangle and quickly prescribing a structural change demonstrates the therapist's ability to have an impact on the family. Such early intervention can enhance the therapist's credibility and engage the family at an early stage in the therapy. (Of course this should be done only after the therapist pays sufficient attention to developing a relationship with the family members and listening to their definition of the problem.)

Thinking about triangles keeps therapists focused on process and helps them to avoid getting mired in the minutiae of content or the morass of dyadic conflict. Suppose, for example, two parents are arguing about whether they should allow their 15-year-old daughter to date. Dealing with the triangle—mother taking the daughter's side against father's objections to unsupervised dates—keeps the therapy focused on what really matters—the relationships among the three of them.

The mistake is to allow the therapy to be detoured (as the family was) into the question of "the truth" about whether a 15-year-old ought to date. That is, dealing with the structure and process of the relationships among the three people will put on the table the alliance between mother and daughter and father's outside position. Dealing with the relationships matters more than talking as if there were some age at which parents should allow all young people to date.

It is important to keep in mind that, no matter what psychotherapeutic model a therapist uses, the problem a patient or couple or family walks in with is less important than the relationship obstacles that keep them from working to resolve it. In this regard, solution-oriented therapists may get too narrowly focused on patients' problem-maintaining behaviors or their unhelpful narrative constructions. Multigenerational therapists may wander aimlessly through extended family fields, never getting to the point. Triangles offer an organizing focus that helps therapists avoid letting their concentration get too narrow or too broad.

Working on triangles helps to promote a different kind of relationship movement in the family. Once movement begins that is different from the old, homeostatic movement, the therapist gets new avenues of access to the family's emotional system. Focusing on triangles in therapy isn't intended to avoid problems in individuals and dyads. On the contrary, clearing away or shifting the triangles allows us to see individual and dyadic problems more easily, more clearly, and in less time, and to deal with them more efficiently. For example, as mother moves back from her daughter, perhaps her depression comes to the surface now that her involvement with her daughter no longer masks it. As father struggles to deal directly with his daughter, the fact that they have never had a truly personal relationship becomes clear. As child tries to restore the old pattern, the child's fears and dependence, previously unacknowledged, appear. In addition, the problems in each dyad become clearer, and relevant unresolved problems in the extended family show up.

These dyadic and family problems emerge from the experiences of the people going through the process of restructuring the triangles. They aren't interpretations made by the therapist. Patients actually experience their own feelings. They are less apt to hear problems and feelings they have actually experienced merely as intellectual ideas coming from a therapist. They are more apt to lead to change, since feelings change by experience.

Thinking about relationship triangles can provide a structure for coaching a patient who wants to improve his or her adaptive level of functioning in a relationship or a system. For instance, Leslie P. was a woman who worried about every aspect of her children's lives and with whom she had always had an overly close and overinvolved relationship. Her son, Carl, was married, and he and his wife had recently had a baby boy. Leslie was aware that Carl's wife, Betsy, while always friendly, was nervous about Leslie's closeness to Carl and her tendency to interfere. The therapist coached Leslie to stay warm and connected but to give Carl and Betsy plenty of room. She phoned regularly but didn't visit for 4 weeks after Betsy and the baby came home from the hospital. When she did visit, Carl let her know that he felt hurt by the infrequency of her visits, but a week later Betsy called and invited Leslie to join her for lunch and to see a play in New York.

Working with triangles is an extremely effective way of overriding homeostasis. Triangle work helps people get "uncaught" from the repetitive, predictable patterns of behavior they engage in even though those patterns don't work, and people know they don't work. Triangles stabilize such patterns by allowing them to be repeated over and over without ending the relationships (and without forcing them to change). Having a third person (or thing) to focus arguments and resentments on sustains the illusion that the real problem between them is that third party. If the disagreement between two people about the third party seems insuperable, the two continue to fight about it in the same way as always.

Detriangling breaks the patterns and gives people new behavioral options. George F. was a 39-year-old man, never married, who presented with the problem that he couldn't "make a commitment." His live-in girlfriend kept giving him ultimatums about marriage, and he kept putting her off. She threatened to leave; he agreed to get engaged; she stayed; he never proposed; she threatened to leave again. The third point of the triangle here was an idealized woman, who seemed to have many of his mother's qualities, though George denied this. "I love my mother, but she's a dingbat, and I could never live with anyone like her." An interlocking triangle was with George's mother's longtime boyfriend. He didn't live with her, traveled a great deal by himself, and, according to George, did pretty much what he wanted while still being "a great guy." George's mother made no demands on this man and seemed quite satisfied with the kind of life she had with him.

George's inability to make a commitment doesn't make nearly as much sense if we view it outside the context of triangles. In therapy based on the model of transference, the therapist might allow dependency to build up in the therapeutic context. When the therapist doesn't deliver on the patient's need for, say, phone calls between sessions, and the patient gets angry, the therapist would make the interpretation that his mother never met the patient's needs for attention and nurturing. In a supportive counseling approach, the therapist might deal with George's dependence on his mother by urging him to separate from her—to see and talk to her less, for example. If we see George's problem in a triangular context, however, the picture is different. George is always moving *away* from his mother toward women, and, when he gets close to one, moving away from her toward the "idealized woman." The emotional process in the triangle is centered on George's denial of his dependence (on his mother and on the women he gets close to). From this viewpoint, it makes sense for therapy to get George to move *toward* his mother. If he works on creating a more adult, one-on-one relationship with his mother, and allows the dependency to emerge and manages it, he may be freed up enough from being caught in this triangle to have an adult relationship with another woman.

Knowing about triangles, being familiar with how they work, and having a repertoire of interventions for exploring and resolving them are invaluable weapons in a therapist's armamentarium, no matter what the therapist's theoretical orientation. Whenever you look carefully at cases that don't respond to treatment or seem stuck, look for a triangle you haven't seen yet. Whether the treatment is systems therapy, psychodynamic therapy, medical treatment, or some combination, you'll find that defining and modifying the relationship triangles surrounding the symptom bearer or the relationship conflict are essential to therapeutic progress.

THE CLINICAL CENTRALITY OF TRIANGLES

The clinical relevance of relationship triangles is based on six factors. Lasting success in therapy usually depends on some resolution of the central triangles surrounding the presenting problem. Picture the following case. A married couple, Mary and John D., developed creeping distance in the relationship over time, partly from his silence and her need to express everything. Mary drew closer to their children and John ended up in the outsider position in that triangle. The outsider position produced feelings of loss and loneliness in him, with difficulty in concentrating, loss of energy, oversleeping, and overeating. His down mood became a mild clinical depression (*factor number one: triangles promote the development of symptoms in the individual*). John wasn't in enough difficulty to motivate anyone in the family to seek therapy. He gradually started to alternate between sulking in his withdrawal and depression and moving toward Mary in angry conflict over the triangular issue of how to raise the children. All this behavior manifested itself when he really wanted more love and attention from her and equal primacy with the children (*factor number two: triangles support the chronicity of symptoms in an individual and of conflict in a relationship*).

Much of the trouble in John and Mary's marriage began when they were first married. Mary had great difficulty separating from her father and making her attachment to John the primary one in her life. Once they had children, she got overly attached to them, too, leaving John in the outside position in both triangles. John, on the other hand, had never dealt with his mother's emotional intensity, and so he had cut off from her and had clung to Mary as his emotional lifeline. There were underlying problems of Mary's attachment to her father, placing him on a pedestal and allowing no room in her heart for her husband. John's failure to develop a mature relationship with his mother created an additional layer of difficulty. If the family doesn't recognize these complexities, the issue may get defined as Mary being too lenient with the children and John being too strict. Then the family and the therapist don't identify or address the underlying toxic emotional difficulties (*factor number three: triangles work against the resolution of toxic or conflictual issues in an individual or a relationship*).

John isolated himself from his children, Mary took refuge in her closeness with them, and the parent–child relations became fixed in distance and over closeness. The marital relationship was fixed in conflict (*factor number four: triangles block the functional evolution of a relationship over time*). The therapist found Mary's sympathetic situation more understandable than John's strict one but didn't want to side with one or the other. If the therapist has no knowledge of triangles, she or he may try to get the parents to agree on a mutual approach to the children. This will result in an endless series of compacts between the parents to handle one situation after another by agreement. The situations will be endless, and the agreements will be poorly operated and forgotten. Therapy will continue until all members become exhausted or run out of money (*factor number five: triangles can create or support the therapeutic impasse*).

Both John and Mary were caught in primary parental triangles in their families of origin and never got free enough from them to form their own relationship. Thus the relationship difficulties in their families of origin got displaced downward onto the marriage, and John and Mary are caught in in-law triangles. Once they have children, the conflict in the marriage got displaced downward onto the children, and the spouses became caught in triangles with their children. The way they were caught in these triangles drove their behavior. They didn't have any autonomy or control over that behavior, and the triangles set the behavior in concrete (*factor number six: triangles get people "caught," depriving them of options*).

The Mechanism of Symptom Activation

Triangles promote the development of symptoms in the individual. Being caught in a triangle is stressful and kindles feelings of helplessness and hopelessness. For example, a child drawn into a triangle because of his sensitivity to emotional upset in his mother internalizes her emotional arousal and begins to underachieve in school and isolate from his friends. An adolescent in developmental turmoil deranges the already shaky truce in his parents' dysfunctional relationship. Triangles refortify the fragile bond by joining the parents in concern for and criticism of him. His response is to feel angry and justified in stealing the family car. A 52-year-old woman dealing with decades of pressure and criticism from her husband and mother feels the noose tighten when her 75-year-old mother comes to live with them. Her frustration and hopelessness over the situation trigger an episode of clinical depression. (Sometimes, however, being caught in a triangle doesn't feel stressful. The wife who feels great about her new affair and the adult child who feels special when his mother complains to him about his father are examples. Eventually, the negative consequences of this willing complicity in being caught in a triangle will show up and feel stressful.)

A person emotionally trapped in a triangle is likely, by virtue of being trapped, to suffer some loss of function. Being caught in a triangle arouses your emotional reactivity to the point where the reactivity constrains your behavior, and you can't imagine any options. Consider, for example, a little girl whose mother develops an anxious attachment to her in response to her husband's distance. As a result the father then becomes very critical of the girl. In response to her position in the triangle, the child may refuse to go to school, or her asthma may get much worse. The intervention here would be to get the father to decrease his level of criticism and move toward his daughter to spend relationship time with her (*not* fixing-her time). Simultaneously, the mother can be encouraged to focus less on her daughter and more on other, neglected areas of her own life. Perhaps she needs to narrow the distance between herself and her own mother. As the triangle shifts, the marital issues may emerge, and treatment can then be directed at them. In any event, working on the triangle at least frees the child and provides relief from her symptom.

The Chronicity of Symptoms

Triangles support the chronicity of symptoms in an individual and of conflict in a relationship. A 48-year-old executive named Bob M. was passed over for a promotion at work, and he became irritable at home, more demanding of sexual attention from Terry, his wife, and much more easily wounded. The loss had activated a mild depression. Terry, anxious about their financial well-being, started to avoid sex, especially in the face of Bob's irritability and babyish behavior. She withdrew from him and looked for a job to provide security in case he were to lose his job. Then Bob felt justified in starting an affair with his divorced neighbor who drove to work with him every day. As long as the milk and honey of the extramarital affair was available Bob wouldn't face his performance at work, his depression over the lost promotion, the conflict and sexual problems in his marriage that preceded the affair. Four years later, the problems were chronic and remained camouflaged. Once symptoms have appeared, or conflict has begun, being caught in a triangle heightens stress. Stress is a pivotal factor in the persistence of symptoms and conflict.

Symptoms in an individual or relationship, which might otherwise be amenable to management or even change, sometimes become entrenched and resistant to direct intervention. Often when this happens it is because the therapy left unaddressed a relationship triangle. For example, a middle-aged woman had a depression that did not respond to trials of several medications. It stayed intractable as long as both her husband and her mother were allied in defining her as sick and trying to get her to "pull herself up by her bootstraps." In working with this couple, the therapist made the alliance between husband and mother-in-law explicit. This put the wife's reaction to it on the table, and the therapist coached the husband in how to take a different position in the triangle. Shifting the structure and changing the process in the triangle addressed the underlying cause of the woman's depression. If medication is prescribed now to help alleviate the symptoms of depression, the problem is less likely to recur than if medication had been employed without addressing the relationship imbalances that led to the depression (or exacerbated it once it was in place).

The Resolution of Toxic or Conflictual Issues

Triangles work against the resolution of toxic or conflictual issues in an individual or a relationship. Consider the case of Bob and Terry. None of the problems between them had been touched. Without the stabilizing effect of the extramarital affair, the problems would have become more visible and have demanded attention. Triangles are a stabilizing distraction.

The Functional Evolution of a Relationship

A triangle can, and very often does, allow the relationship system to continue without change and without resolving issues that need to be resolved. For example, an extramarital affair makes it "unnecessary" to address the sexual immaturity of a couple in which one spouse is sexually demanding and the other sexually constricted. The lover is meeting the demands of the spouse having the affair, and that takes the pressure off the constricted spouse, who therefore feels less pressured. If the therapist persuades the spouse having the affair to end it, the sexual issues are likely to become explicit and can be dealt with in treatment. If the therapist persuades the unfaithful spouse to stop the affair, that person will experience three reactions: feelings of loss of the relationship and the emotional and sexual perks that went along with it, anger at the spouse for having to suffer this loss when the spouse's behavior was the justification for the affair in the first place, and issues of sexual incompatibility that may be driving the distance and the acting out.

A therapist without a knowledge of triangles will get caught into the therapy triangle of being judgmental about the affair or into justifying it based on the betrayed partner's behavior. In either case, the therapist is caught, a new triangle is formed, and the process gets displaced into the therapy triangle instead of involved in dealing with the affair. A triangle can, and very often does, allow the relationship system to continue without change and without resolving issues that need to be resolved.

Triangles block the functional evolution of a relationship over time. They keep relationships frozen in the same old quarrels and issues and don't allow relationships to grow and change as circumstances change and as the life cycle progresses. Bob's extramarital affair had put the marital relationship on hold for 4 years. Because the affair hadn't stopped, and Bob and Terry hadn't dealt with the underlying problems and their fallout, the evolutionary maturing of their relationship remained arrested. Their marriage began to deteriorate to the chronic distance of an emotional divorce. The next developmental crisis might cause the final fracture of the marriage.

It is natural and desirable that relationships grow and mature over time. As a son or daughter grows up, for instance, his or her relationship with parents should go from childlike dependence to an adult relationship. Triangles can retard this development, as in a triangle where a mother is overly close with her child and father is in the distant position. The relationship between mother and child won't evolve appropriately as the child grows older, and the child may remain infantilized, even as an adult. This adult may come to therapy because of his difficulty in forming romantic attachments. If the therapist thinks that the patient's position in his or her primary parental triangle is at the root of that patient's problem, she or he would coach the patient to shift the triangle. The patient does this by finding ways to move toward the father and to behave in a less childlike way with the mother.

Therapeutic Impasse

Triangles can create or support the therapeutic impasse. An unaddressed triangle is a vehicle for voluntary noncompliance with treatment or is a reason for involuntary noncompliance. When a patient suffering from depression fails to respond to the most sophisticated combination of drugs and psychotherapy, look for a background triangle that you can't easily see. The same is true for a marital conflict that defies intervention. First review to see if the therapist is caught in a triangle with the couple. If not, search for a background triangle that is supporting noncompliance with therapy. (The individual therapist of one or both spouses may be one place to look.)

A therapeutic impasse is most often caused by noncompliance, misdiagnosis, or a mismatch between the patient's abilities and the type of therapy being used. Triangles play a role in creating or supporting the impasse. When therapy is stuck, it can often be unstuck if the therapist stops to look for and work on unresolved triangles. These triangles may be embroiling the patient, blocking the therapy, or both.

When mental health professionals trained in a psychodynamic paradigm are faced with a therapeutic impasse, they think about the patient's defenses, resistance, or problems in the transference. After reviewing these factors, they consider possible countertransference problems. For instance, an analyst might be puzzling over why a 50-year-old woman hasn't yet developed a positive transference in spite of lengthy therapy. The analyst might be speculating that her apparently obsessive curiosity about him is the cause of the problem. This may be the problem, but the problem may be supported by the woman's husband. Perhaps he is suspicious that the therapist is turning his wife against him and insists on knowing the therapist's marital status.

A psychiatrist may be treating a patient with a major clinical depression that isn't responding to antidepressants. The first step is to check that the patient is complying with the prescribed program of treatment. If the patient is compliant, the psychiatrist then searches for a different drug to which the patient might have a better response. In addition, the psychiatrist might profitably check on whether a family member with influence over the patient is negative about medication in general or psychotropic medication in particular. Consider, for example, the case of a 27-year-old married woman with early-morning awakening, loss of appetite and libido, difficulty concentrating, and a preoccupation with thoughts of death and dying. The psychiatrist tried several serotonin reuptake inhibitors without much change. When he asked about the woman's compliance, he found that the patient was "forgetting" to take her medication about three times a week. The physician asked to see the woman's husband and learned that the possibility his wife could become addicted to the medication frightened him, and he told his wife so every day. The psychiatrist educated this man about the biochemical aspects of depression and about how antidepressants work. He explained that depression was at the root of his wife's recent behavior (including loss of libido), and that medication was likely to relieve her symptoms. The husband was relieved and agreed to encourage his wife to comply with the medical regimen. She did, and her symptoms improved markedly within a month.

Getting Caught

Triangles get people "caught," depriving them of options and ensuring that their behavior will continue in the same dysfunctional rut. People can experience therapy triangles as supportive when in fact the only things they are supportive of is the chronicity of the symptoms around which they were formed.

In active triangles, people are never free. Their responses to events are constrained and predictable. They are unable to consider alternatives. Even if they can think of something different to do, they are afraid to risk it. They fear that they or someone else will get hurt or angry with them or leave. Joseph P., a 30-year-old married man in couple therapy, was working hard on controlling his tendency to shout at Linda, his wife. His therapist asked him who else he has shouted at like that, and whether anyone had shouted at him. These questions made it possible for him to link his anger with the feelings he used to get as an adolescent. His mother would complain to him about her life and, he thought, expect him to make it all better. When he couldn't, his mother would act disappointed in him, and he would feel helpless and inadequate. Then he would become withdrawn and rebellious, and his father would yell at him and call him names. When Linda criticized him or made demands on him, he would feel helpless and inadequate all over again, and get furious with her "for making him feel that way."

Joseph agreed that he had never found a way to deal with his mother's complaints and demands so that he was disconnected from them while staying in touch with her. Every time she complained or demanded, he tried to fix things or reassure her that everything would be all right. Inevitably, he failed. He then got angry with his mother for "making him feel inadequate." In therapy, Joseph couldn't think of any other way to approach these situations (except to avoid his mother). When the therapist suggested various experiments to him, he found himself unable to try them in the field, although they "sounded terrific" to him in the therapy room. One problem Joseph had with these experiments was that he expected *not to have* the uncomfortable feelings he usually got with his mother if he tried something different with her. As soon as he started to feel uncomfortable, he assumed that the experiment had failed even before he tried it. He had hoped that having a different plan would prevent those feelings. The reality is that the *feelings* will continue to come for a while. The first step for Joseph in getting uncaught is to manage his feelings and not be determined in his *behavior* by them. This will insure that his emotions won't drive him into a set of predictable actions. The next step for Joseph is to monitor what happens inside himself when he refrains from getting angry with his mother. Is there a new feeling, a vacuum, or what? This kind of self-control and raised consciousness is the beginning of change. The next step is to observe what happens to Joseph's mother when he behaves differently. It's predictable that she will escalate her efforts to bring Joseph back into his usual pattern of behavior. If he can get past that, if he can see what is happening and hold his position without showing his resentment, eventually his feelings will change too. At that point he will be detriangled, and he will have a much better chance of controlling his anger at his wife.

CHAPTER THREE

Addressing Triangles in Therapy

In his teaching about clinical intervention based on family systems theory, Guerin describes a model of therapy based on the assumption that developmental and situational stress trigger anxiety and depression in the individual. This state of emotional arousal often results in behavior patterns that produce conflict in relationships and support dysfunction in the individuals. This process inevitably activates surrounding relationship triangles and becomes embedded in them. These triangles in turn reinforce pathology in the individuals and conflict in their relationships. A husband who finds his job of 20 years threatened by the arrival of a new employee from a competitor becomes irritable, short-tempered, distracted, and distant during his evenings and weekends at home. His wife, frightened by his inner turmoil and aware of his usual unwillingness to talk about it, begins a predictable series of solicitous behaviors directed toward him. Such behavior further irritates the husband and decreases the likelihood of his talking about the threat to his job. Hurt by the rejection that she feels, the wife retreats to help her son with his homework only to find her husband already there, criticizing her son's study habits and school performance. The triangles multiply, the individual dysfunction continues, and the situational stress is never addressed and dealt with.

Psychotherapy based on this model attempts to find the vulnerable and injured strands of the individuals and their relationships, disentangle them from the snarls of their interlocking triangles, and weave them back together with stronger relationships between individuals who are functioning better and are more autonomous. Adding the relationship triangle to the therapist's conceptual framework and working on triangles in therapy are essential for successful work on both individual and relationship problems. Connecting individual and relationship problems to the multiple triangles that surround and entangle them is one major factor that distinguishes our therapeutic model from others. This means that therapy becomes a lattice work in which the focus moves freely back and forth among the inner lives of the individuals, the dyadic personal relationships those individuals are in, and the relationship triangles that surround and entangle those dyads.

The following cases all illustrate the interplay among individual factors, the interpersonal relationships, and the triangles that surround those relationships. Each case came to therapy with a different original focus. One presented as an individual dysfunction. The second was a marital problem without explicit triangles, and the third was a marital case with explicit triangles. The fourth was a child-focused case. In spite of their differences, all four required attention to the entire web of individuals, dyads, and triangles.

Connie B. was a 50-year-old single banker who came to therapy with complaints of depression and panic attacks. She found herself crying a lot, not sleeping, unable to concentrate on her job, and feeling hopeless about ever getting better. She described her panic as coming on without warning in a variety of settings, such as work, shopping, and driving, and producing choking sensations, palpitations, dizziness, faintness, and a terrifying sense of impending doom. Between attacks she lived in fear, always worrying that another attack would come.

Connie had always lived with her parents, and she and her mother had continued to share the family home after Connie's father died. She had been involved for 15 years with an older divorced man who lived in a distant city. She had recently found evidence that this man had been unfaithful: pictures of another woman in his bedroom, wearing only a bra and panties. Connie had been reluctant to confront her friend, terrified that their relationship would end and she would end up alone.

Connie B. came into therapy as an "individual" case, with a clinical depression, complicated by panic attacks requiring medication and psychotherapy. The briefest of interviews, however, revealed that these individual symptoms were related to a relationship problem with her long-term boyfriend. That relationship problem, in turn, was entangled in an obvious triangle, her lover's affair with another woman. Another, more subtle, triangle was also an important ingredient in the mixture. Connie's mother was the most important influence in Connie's life. The therapist thought that the mother–daughter fusion had been intensified by her father's death and by unresolved issues in Connie's primary parental triangle. This fusion played a major role in Connie's panic attacks and in the way her relationship with her boyfriend developed. Connie's case called for a contextualization of her symptoms and an understanding of their evolution. Ideally, therefore, therapy would include not only medication aimed at her symptoms, but also psychotherapy dealing with the underlying emotional forces (individual, dyadic, *and* triangular) driving those symptoms. Unfortunately, Connie was unwilling to explore these issues and left therapy after getting relief from the depression and panic.

In leaving when she did, Connie was typical of many people who come to therapy, get symptom relief, and leave without engaging in the work necessary for long-term change. This is a reality in the practice of psychotherapy, and it raises the question of how a therapist should deal with it. You can only deal with people leaving when they decide to by applying as much of your model as fits the case and fits the patient's choices about treatment. Always, however, the therapist ought to check on whether an active triangle is driving the early termination. For example, in a transference-based model, an early termination might be the result of a triangle consisting of the therapist, the patient, and some internalized object. The therapist might be trying to move the patient toward an object that the patient is not ready to deal with, and the patient leaves because of that. In a model like ours, which works to reduce transference, the therapist needs to be alert to the possibility that a triangle may be determining the therapist's response to therapy's ending. Is your decision to disagree with a patient's decision based on your being caught in a therapy triangle (you're being overresponsible about keeping her in therapy and preventing her from moving back to her family, which she's ready to do) or is it based on a principle of stating clearly your own opinion? Is your decision to allow a patient to leave without disagreement based on a therapy triangle (you're too distant from the patient because there's something about her that irritates you or makes you anxious) or on your principle of always showing respect for a patient's decision? Is a patient's desire to end therapy based on the belief that he or she has gotten what it was he or she wanted, or is there an active therapy triangle (maybe you've gotten caught between the patient and a family member you've come to think of as villainous) that is making this patient uncomfortable and pushing him or her out?

Phil and Jeanne C. were a couple in their early 40s with two adolescent children who came to therapy with complaints of marital conflict. They were alienated from one another, with little communication and no mutual affection, lobbing critical grenades at each other about real and perceived grievances. Both dated the deterioration of their relationship from an automobile accident that Phil had had 4 years before. He hadn't found steady employment since, and Jeanne had been forced to go back to work.

The couple described many problems between them that centered on money. For example, Phil hadn't paid the mortgage for many months without telling Jeanne, and she only found out about it when the bank began foreclosure. The hottest issue then however, was the behavior of their daughter, Sara, age 12. Jeanne said that Sara was out of control and that nothing they did could get her to "behave like a human being." Jeanne was finally ready to consider Ritalin in spite of her longstanding opposition to it. Phil attributed Sara's problems to a "lack of consistency" around discipline on Jeanne's part. Each spouse blamed the other for the problem.

Although Phil and Jeanne C. came in as a marital case, in the first weeks of treatment they found it nearly impossible to stay focused on their relationship. No matter what questions the therapist asked them, their replies centered either on the problems they were having with their daughter or on Phil's problems with work. Their answers always had Jeanne accusing Phil of irresponsibility and inconsiderateness and Phil defending himself. The treatment plan for this case called first for circling in on the marital relationship. Jeanne needed to tone down her criticism of Phil; Phil needed to stop defending himself and to raise his level of functioning. The second part of the plan was to modify the parental triangle with Sara by shifting each partner's part in the process. Third, therapy had to discover the important triangles that interlock with the Sara triangle and work on them. Unlike Connie, whose symptoms required contextualization, Phil and Jeanne came in with a multifocused problem requiring them to stop projecting and get self-focused.

Stan and Maryellen D., a couple in their late 20s, married for 4 years, sought therapy complaining that they rarely had sex anymore. Both were bright, successful people who manifested no signs of individual pathology, but both were wondering whether their young marriage was already dying. Stan said that he often felt "in the middle" between his mother and Maryellen, who were constantly criticizing each other. It seemed to him that they pressured him to take sides. Maryellen reported that her mother-in-law wanted to be in control of their lives and was always telling them what to do.

Certain triangles occur most commonly in particular developmental stages. For instance, in early marriage, the in-law triangle is the most common; at the birth of a baby or when children reach adolescence, the child-centered triangle is likely to be active and intense. Stan and Maryellen were a young couple in the early stages of their marriage, and it was the in-law triangle that they needed to negotiate in order to connect with one another. Who would be more important to Stan, his mother or his wife? Who would have more influence over him? Primacy of attachment and of influence are powerful issues early in a marriage. Thus, the therapist planned to move the triangle by shifting both spouses' participation in it: Stan could move toward his mother in a more adult way; Maryellen could get herself emotionally neutral about her mother-in-law. When they had made progress in the triangle, the therapist could deal with any residual sexual issues.

Kevin E. was an 11-year-old boy brought to therapy by his mother because he was getting deficiency reports in his academic subjects. He was the youngest of three boys, with a 12-year gap between him and his next older brother. He had an overly close relationship with his mother, Anne, 50, who was in the middle of treatment for breast cancer. Kevin's father, Paul, also 50, was in the distant position from Kevin and from Anne. No one was talking about Anne's cancer, except the logistics of her treatment. Kevin's view of his problem was that he was a "nerd" who didn't belong, and he desperately wanted to be more popular.

Clearly Kevin had temperament problems and developmental dilemmas to deal with on his own. Yet the struggle going on his family was making these issues worse. The family wasn't facing Anne's illness and possible death. There was a chronic triangle in which Anne was overly close to Kevin and Paul was too distant. Kevin had been born shortly after Anne's father died, making him special to Anne. On the other hand, he was a child very much unlike what Paul, a star athlete in college, hoped for from a son of his.

Treatment in this case called for work on all three levels. Individual sessions with Kevin focused on play time with the therapist to consolidate the connection between them. The therapist asked Kevin to bring Nintendo and Sega games to the office to help the therapist get better at video games. Kevin also reviewed the seating chart of his classroom and how his relationships were improving with key class-mates. Together Kevin and the therapist would review whether there had been an increase or a decrease in his "nerdy" behavior over the 2 weeks between sessions. As Kevin felt safe enough to talk about his progress or lack of it, the therapist felt that the timing was right to open discussions about Kevin's paternal grandfather's advancing Alzheimer's disease and his mother's cancer.

In alternating biweekly sessions with Kevin's parents, the therapist encouraged Paul to spend more relationship time with his son, doing activities of his son's choosing. He also coached Paul to remain open to any references from Kevin to Paul's father and to Anne's illness. Anne was coached to focus her efforts on healing her cancer and was offered either individual, couple, or family sessions to help with the emotional fallout from her focus on the cancer when she felt ready. The therapist modeled frank and sensitive discussions about Anne's cancer, and coached them to have such discussions at home. The long-term triangle needed to be restructured so that Kevin and Paul would have more of a relationship and Kevin's relationship with his mother would be less intense. It was a matter of clinical judgment how all three of these issues were dealt with over time, whether all three people should come to therapy at the same time, or whether some issues should be discussed in pairs or with individuals alone. It's best to keep all options open at any given time. In certain situations, having a separate therapist for each person may be advisable.

The best therapy connects the individual experience of anxiety and depression, the dyadic process of relationship conflict, and the triangles surrounding both of them. Weaving all these threads together in therapy requires a level of familiarity and comfort with the clinical forms and functions of triangles. This includes a knowledge of the concept, a facility with thinking about triangles to be able to find them, a facility with working triangles in the systems that come to therapy, and an ability to stay out of triangles as a therapist. In what follows, we hope to demystify relationship triangles and help you learn to recognize and deal with them in a wide range of individual and family problems.

SELF-FOCUS

It is a natural emotional reflex for each of us to look outside of ourselves for the cause of our pain and discomfort. Our everyday conversations with one another betray this tendency. "You made me angry." "If it weren't for your failure as a parent, I could do anything." Part of being a grown-up entails developing ease at stepping up and assuming responsibility for one's own emotions and the relationship behavior that these emotions drive. If any of us fails at this key developmental task, that person is doomed to a life of angry, resentful victimhood. As psychotherapy tries to be supportive, it must be careful not to step over the line of enabling a self-righteous victimhood. An important antidote to this therapeutic trap is to emphasize the importance of being able to self-focus—that is, to work at seeing the parts of ourselves that contribute significantly to our own pain and our relationship discomfort.

It is more usual than not for us humans to see clearly what is the *other* person's part in a relationship problem. We view ourselves as well-motivated folks who somehow end up in relationship dilemmas when other people screw up. If only *they* could be different, more sensitive, then no problem!

With chronic farsightedness, we accept without questions the way we ourselves are and believe that if we are difficult at times we can't help it. The other side of the equation—our spouses, our children, our parents, our bosses, and coworkers—*could* alter their behavior if they really wanted to. We, who are doing our very best, lose sight of our side of the equation, especially in those everyday relationships where we have long ago slipped into automatic responses. Blind with the pain of our relationship struggles, we can't see our own piece of the problem. All we can see is the part of the problem in the one we love, who to our puzzlement seems at times to act like the enemy.

For the work on relationship triangles to make sense to people, therapists need to reinforce their patients' ability to recognize that blaming the other for the problem without understanding their own contribution to the problem continues the relationship dysfunction and gives people no leverage to change their own misery. Instead, they place all the power in the other. It's the therapist's task to help people see that they can change their own part in a process and so change their lives. Interaction is like a play—everyone involved plays *some* part. If you're not playing Romeo, then you're playing Juliet, or Signor Capulet, or Signora Montague. If therapy doesn't make the shift to people taking responsibility for themselves, conflict and dysfunction will continue and even intensify.

Self-focus is the ability to see a relationship problem as a result not only of the other person's limitation but also of one's own. For example, in a marriage where the husband is often silent and distant, his part in the problem is obvious (at least to his wife). Still, what part might she be playing? Is she a good listener or does she interrupt and criticize him when he does talk? Is his experience of her one in which he feels safe to say what he thinks? Or does he think that she'll get upset at whatever he says, and then he'll have to deal with that—one of his least favorite things? If an elderly mother is still telling her middle-aged daughter how to live her life, could the daughter have a part in the problem? Has she been unable to handle the assault of her mother's anxiety, and gently to neutralize the cycles of conflict in their relationship, or if necessary even to take a strong "I" position with her mother? "You know, mother, the more you tell me what to do, the more I find myself doing the opposite, and resenting you for the unasked-for advice."

Encouraging self-focus in therapy isn't a way to let the other person off the hook but, rather, a way to discourage blaming. Blaming just feeds the reactivity in a relationship. Self-focus isn't an attempt to release others from responsibility; it's a way for people to have more control in their own lives. It's a way of thinking that gives people more options for movement than an angry helpless victim has. For example, having a son who's drug-addicted is very difficult. A parent feels responsible and angry that the child is wasting his young life. Obviously the son is dysfunctional and has intense—even life-threatening—problems. The parent, who might be doing quite well in the rest of her life, still needs to self-focus. What is her bottom line with her son? How does she deal with the helplessness she feels when she begins to see her impotence to save him and to "get him off drugs"?

Learning to see one's own role in a twosome can be hard. Learning to see one's own role in a *triangle* can be even more difficult. Maybe that's because two-against-one can increase a person's feelings of victimization. Maybe it's because some triangles can be below the surface and difficult to see. It's only when the therapist has elicited the triangle and made it explicit that it becomes clear why a person is caught and doesn't know why. Sometimes it's hard to see our own part in a triangle because we're not used to thinking about triangles.

The ability to see one's self and behavior in the context of a relationship is tremendously important to the successful alteration of one's position in a triangle. It's important to learn not to blame so that one isn't run by reactivity. People can think better and more clearly if their emotions aren't in an uproar. With less reactivity and less emotionality, people can begin to see how they might change. Learning to track our own reactions and behavior can interrupt knee-jerk responses that help perpetuate a problem.

Ellen S. came to therapy complaining of depression. She was also furious with her husband, whom she blamed for her unhappiness. When she wasn't blaming her husband, she focused on her son, whom she found manipulating and selfish, or her mother, whom she labeled narcissistic, or her father-in-law, whom she saw as the cause of her husband's insensitivity. The only person in her life Ellen seemed pleased with was her 7-year-old daughter, whom she was so eager to see at the end of the day that she *always* picked her up at school. Picking up one's child at school every day by itself has no particular significance, but in Ellen's case, her overinvolvement with her daughter and her fury with her husband and son made for some intense triangles. Once the therapist could help Ellen see that the only person she could change was herself, and that her anger and helplessness with others were fueling her depression, she could get interested in what *she* could do to change. She focused on herself, stopped criticizing others, and took responsibility for her own happiness.

People don't always come to us thinking that everything is someone else's fault. Sometimes they come to therapy in a self-blaming position. "I'm all wrong. I need to change everything. It's because of me that things are so bad." This is a *pseudo*-self-focus, and it isn't helpful. If therapists dig a little underneath its surface, usually they find real anger and outrage, or the patient is so depressed that the therapist must address the depression before any triangle work is done.

Whether therapists are dealing with blaming, helplessness, or self-deprecation, people's lack of self-focus is going to affect the outcome of their work. The more intense the blaming, the less the ability to focus on self, the more severe will be the implicit or explicit conflict in people's relationships. One way to assess the degree of self-focus is to ask each person to draw up a list of his or her limitations that contribute to the relationship problem. This helps when the individual insists that the other person *really* is 95% responsible for the problem. The therapist can concentrate on the 5% the individual admits may be his or her part and so begin the work of self-focus.

It also needs to be said that a formidable impediment to increasing self-focus in our patients is the development of a therapy triangle (see p. 145 ff.). When we're caught in the middle rather than being detached enough to be useful and effective, then the people we're supposed to help will have little chance of developing enough self-focus to change their lives. A therapy triangle is one good indication that *somebody*—the therapist? the patient?—has lost self-focus.

WHAT A TRIANGLE IS NOT

Triangles are different from threesomes. A group of three isn't necessarily a triangle. The distinction is an important one. People can become so overly sensitive to the existence of triangles that they see any group of three people as a triangle, or any viewpoint about a third person as a triangle.

A threesome can be broken down into three simultaneous twosomes—that is, three interconnected twosomes that simultaneously are in some kind of distant (relatively uninvolved) or a close, intensely involved relationship. All three members can interact with each other, one-on-one, depending on what the situation calls for. They have options. They can choose to be involved or uninvolved and to vary their involvement so that it isn't necessarily reactive and predictable (such as always being angry or always being sympathetic). Each member of the threesome can take an honest, diplomatic "I" position with any other member of the threesome without trying to change the other two or trying to impose that position on the others. Each member can allow the other two to have their own relationship, work out their own problems, and enjoy their particular pleasures, without interfering to "make peace," to instigate conflict, or to side with one against the other. It is characteristic of a threesome that each person in a threesome has a sense of freedom and an ability to focus on self rather than looking to see where the others stand before taking his or her own stand—in other words, being determined by them (see Table 3.1).

An example of the child-centered family, where the problem appears in the child, may show the difference between a triangle and a threesome. In this kind of clinical presentation, the typical triangle is mother and child overly close with the father in the distant position. When a therapist spots this configuration, it doesn't necessarily indicate anything more than a potential triangle. In the absence of a critical level of reactivity that determines behavior, it remains a threesome (although potentially a triangle). It may only be an episode in the life of the family in which the father has a real but temporary disruption in his relationship with his child. It may be that the parents have a real difference of opinion about how to deal with the child,

TABLE 3.1. Comparison of Threesomes and Triangles

Threesomes	Triangles
Each twosome can interact one-on-one.	Each twosome's interaction is tied to the behavior of the third person.
Each person has options for his or her behavior.	Each person is tied to reactive forms of behavior.
Each person can take "I" positions without trying to change the other two.	No one can take an "I" position without needing to change the others.
Each person can allow the other two to have their own relationship without interference.	Each person gets involved in the relationship between the other two.
Self-focus is possible and the usual situation.	No self-focus in anyone, and everyone is constantly focused on the other two.

and the father is staying out of the mother and child twosome because she was there first and is handling the problem. On the other hand, if this pattern becomes consistent and predictable, fixed over time, driven and maintained by anger, hurt, and resentment, then it becomes a triangle. As we watch a threesome–triangle evolve over time, the difference becomes clear.

To detriangle the child-focused case, we have mother (if she is the overinvolved parent) pull back from the child and turn the child over to the distant parent, in this case the father. The process that follows is unvarying. First, the mother feels relieved by having the frustrating burden of the child removed. Then she begins to feel depressed, angry, and empty. The critically important child has been removed from her and given to the undeserving father. As she struggles with these feelings, she grows impatient about the snail's pace at which father is becoming involved with his child. The child, furthermore, reports to her that the father is impossible to deal with or that he's unavailable. The father has trouble moving toward the child and looks to his wife to ask her advice about how he should do this or to get a sense of approval of how he's handling the child. The therapist can literally feel the emotional tension as the triangle struggles from all three positions to prevent detriangling. The homeostatic pressure may be fostered from outside the triangle. For example, the maternal grandmother may criticize her daughter, the mother, for not being more involved with the child. This pattern illustrates the production of interlocking triangles.

If the parents hold on, the child's behavior gets better. As this happens there is usually a deterioration in the marital relationship. The interpersonal problem between husband and wife *emerges by itself.* The therapist doesn't have to dig for it and usually shouldn't. The bedrock of triangles, the avoidance of problems in a twosome, emerges, and the parents report that "things are getting worse" though the child's behavior has improved.

The process in a threesome would be entirely different. The mother can pull back from her child with little difficulty, and the father can easily engage the child. The twosomes are allowed to develop and work their way out of problems. Although one parent may differ from the other, there is a confidence that the other parent will succeed, or, if not, will make the necessary changes. The twosomes form easily, and the third party recognizes that he or she has legitimate business with each of the other two, but no business in that third relationship—the one between the other two. The father can punish the child and mother can stay out of it even if she disagrees with her husband. All can respect the rule that the first parent on the scene handles the problem with the child unless it's in an area that they've agreed belongs to the other. Likewise, all agree that the child is out of line if he or she tries to triangle by going to a parent for a different decision after getting an unfavorable one from the other parent. In other words, the one who tries to triangle is assumed to be acting dysfunctionally. Generally, in a threesome (as opposed to an active triangle) there is usually one person present at any given time who is listening and feeling, but not reacting or taking an active part in the transaction.

Like everything else in life, the triangle is obvious in its grossest form. In the gray area it isn't always clear if there is a triangle or a threesome present. It may have to be observed over time, since they both operate on a continuum, and a threesome can slide into a triangle under stress and then back to a threesome again. When the action is consistent and predictable around a certain issue or problem, it's likely to be a triangle. When there is no choice of response, then the process is reactive and almost certainly triangular.

Just in case things aren't complicated enough, it's possible for one person to be in a threesome, but for the other two to be in a triangle by *using* the third person as a triangular member without his or her active participation. This happens a lot in therapy. For example, the therapist asks the couple not to discuss their situation on the trip home. Yet one will say to the other that the therapist really agreed with him and nailed the other one as the problem. Then they argue about the therapist. The twosome is using as the third leg of the triangle what they *want* the therapist's position to be and not the actual therapist or his or her position or instructions. The experienced therapist will try to neutralize such behavior by responding to it with process questions. For example, "How was the trip home after the last appointment? Did you both agree about whose side I was on?"

Some people are so scared of triangles that they refuse to talk about anyone who isn't in the room. This denies one of humanity's universal dysfunctions, the desire to gossip. Gossip isn't attractive, but it isn't necessarily dysfunctional. *It may simply be gossip.* It's important to remember that the essence of a triangle is to lower anxiety in the individual and tension in the twosome by shifting to the discussion of a third person or issue. Gossip, on the other hand, is the discussion of trifling, often baseless, rumors usually of a personal, sensational, intimate, negative nature, out of a desire to satisfy curiosity, to make one feel better by putting others down, or to avoid looking at self (an avoidance of self but not necessarily of tension in a twosome). Being in a triangle as opposed to a threesome is experienced internally by a sense of anxiety, a falling off of the easy flow of conversation, a wondering about what to say or an uncomfortable silence.

A triangle isn't any gathering of three people. It isn't any gathering where people differ or where the emotional temperature rises. It isn't, except in the most severe cases, a fixed process—always there. In a threesome, there is a fluidity of movement back and forth where patterns are changeable and not predictable. People can change positions, and movement flows in all directions. There is a minimum of assumptions and a maximum of questions to validate that one person has really heard the other. Little is taken for granted, and each person realizes that he or she does not and will never fully know the other. Triangles tend to be limited in the flow of movement, rigid and often very intense in their emotional climate.

An important point about what triangles aren't is that it isn't necessarily a triangle if a person agrees with another and disagrees with a third. That person may be accused of taking sides, and intense negative feelings may be aroused. This may or may not be a triangle, depending on whether the first person bases his or her viewpoint on principle or on feeling. If *A* has a viewpoint that happens to agree with *B* and differ with *C*, *A* is in a triangle if that viewpoint is based on his or her feelings about *B* or *C*. It isn't a triangle if it's based on a belief (right or wrong), a principle that *A* is willing to apply to both *B* and *C* (and indeed him- or herself). *A* might be mistaken, but *A* *isn't* in a triangle. (Of course, that's sometimes a very difficult line to draw—one person's principle may be another's feeling.)

The misunderstanding of this principle often keeps therapists from answering questions, using their extensive experience, and avoiding critical issues of emotional function. All this to "avoid being in a triangle." Therapists, like everyone, need to learn that it's better to get triangled or to triangle than to refuse to be involved and to be safe but ineffective. We all get into triangles. That's to be expected. The real difficulty is being in a triangle, not recognizing it, and continuing endlessly in that same triangle. The fear of being triangled can be as destructive as the self-righteous defense of triangling out of good motives.

People wonder if we ever get out of triangling in our close relationships. From the viewpoint of structure, we can certainly recognize and manage our feelings so that we avoid or reduce the frequency and intensity of the triangles we're involved in. From an emotional point of view, it's questionable whether we can get beyond managing these feelings. It's certainly the work of a lifetime to change feelings inside us that have been present since childhood and may very well remain operational no matter how well we manage them or for how long. Managing our feelings may be the best we can hope for in this process of detriangling. The managed feelings may well remain managed, but we may be saying at the same time that the other isn't managing his or her feelings very well. Is all repression a bad thing? Or is there a difference between knowledgeable, disciplined, and purposeful control of the self and the open, free expression of feelings?

CHAPTER FOUR

The Structure of Relationship Triangles

HOW TO SEE A TRIANGLE

A system is an assemblage of interrelated parts plus the way they function together. The human body illustrates how organic systems work. The *structure* of a single cell in the human body is made up of a cell wall, a cell membrane, and a nucleus with its cytoplasm and important organelles. The *process* going on in the cell is the taking in of nutrients and extrusion of wastes. The structure and process of the cell together serve the *function* of the cell's survival and reproduction. An automobile engine is a familiar example of a mechanical system. An automobile engine is made up of elements such as the carburetor, valves, pistons, spark plugs, and distributor (structure). The parts take in fuel and produce controlled combustion (process), resulting in locomotion (function). Structure, process, and function are elements in all systems, organic, mechanical, and others. Emotional systems are no exception; they, too, involve structure, process, and function. The relationship triangle illustrates the point for emotional systems.

It takes time to see relationship triangles. One sign of a triangle is its repetitive structure. Another is the predictable nature of the process that goes on in a triangle because it's reactive and automatic. Repetition and predictability take time to observe. It's difficult to bring alive the notion of the triangle's interlocking structure, process, and function with the same immediacy as the cell or the automobile engine. One way to do so is to use Thomas Fogarty's[1] notion of the rubber band holding three people together. Imagine three people with a length of rubber band around them. They're prohibited from allowing the rubber band to fall to the ground (perhaps by an unspoken but unbreakable rule). The rubber band creates a *structure* that holds the three people in relationship to one another. The structure limits their *movement.* It forces each of them to compensate for the movement of either or both of the other two to keep the band taut. Maintaining the rubber band so that it doesn't snap or fall to the floor is the reactive *process,* the necessary tension, that requires each individual in the triangle to keep the focus on where the other two people are and on what they're doing. Each individual must move his or her position in reaction to the moves of the other two and can't move freely in reaction to self. The consequence (i.e., *function* or *dysfunction*) of this structure and the accompanying process of the triangle is to stabilize the three relationships and prevent change.

Now picture any two people: spouses, friends, a parent and a child, and notice how the twosome becomes an active triangle. Take Jane F. and her 6-year-old daughter, Jennifer, as an example. The relationship between them exists in what we might call relationship space. The relationship space between the two is a channel within which there is an invisible flow of the emotional energy coming from each person. If Jane, for example, is anxious about her relationship with her husband, Peter, Jennifer may pick up her mother's anxiety, without necessarily knowing what it is about. This absorption of Jane's anxiety will trigger an emotional reaction in Jennifer, which she may convert into symptomatic behavior—for example, the child becomes whiny and demanding. Jane may complain to Peter about the child, and he may join her in disciplining Jennifer. Thus Peter and Jane both become focused on Jennifer and avoid their own relationship and its conflict. This is the point at which emotions activate a triangle. The process appears natural and automatic, but we can track it. The therapist watches one person's emotional arousal (as tension, anxiety, internal conflict, or something similar) feed into a dyad that cannot tolerate that level of emotionality. It is then that the triangle is activated.

In this example, Jane, in a tension-filled dyad (she and her husband) became increasingly anxious and moved toward a third person

---

[1] Fogarty (1975).

(Jennifer) as a refuge. Jane's level of anxiety was picked up by Jennifer (thanks to their fusion), and the child was unable to tolerate it. Jennifer countered via unacceptable behavior (expressed as movement; acting out is a form of distancing), and Jane moved toward her husband for an alliance. Peter joined Jane in the focus on Jennifer, and the triangle was fully activated. The key to following this process is to focus on the movement. That is, rather than getting caught up in the story, the therapist should observe what people are doing with the anxiety flowing through the channel. What direction are they moving in? What or whom are they moving toward or away from in reaction to this flowing anxiety? The triangle serves a *purpose*, functional and/ or dysfunctional. Here, the triangular process between Jane and her daughter serves the (dys)function of avoiding the greater anxiety between Jane and Peter.

Such a case is liable to present as a child-centered problem. The task of the therapist is to modify the *structure* of the triangle by finding a way to move Peter and Jennifer together while helping Jane reduce her overinvolvement with her daughter. This shift in structure through Peter's and Jane's *movement* will probably give symptom relief in short order. It will also reveal the emotional *process* that underlies the triangle, including Jane's anxiety and depression, and the marital distance or conflict. The *function* of the triangle—here, avoidance of that process and of the need to deal with it—will also become clear, at least to the therapist. The family may go away after getting the symptom relief, or they may decide to stay in therapy and deal with the issues that have emerged.

It isn't true that every time parents bring a child to therapy the problem can and will always turn out to be a marital problem, or even an individual problem with one parent. Sometimes the problem is *also* in the child, and sometimes *only* in the child. Brenda T., a 14-year-old, was an example of the former. An accomplished ballerina and actress, she was brought to therapy by her mother, a 40-year-old woman from a wealthy family and married to a successful attorney. Mrs. T. reported that Brenda was "nasty" to her younger brother and sister all the time and refused to eat with the family or participate in any family activities.

The family's recent history included many stressors, not the least of which were Mrs. T.'s surgery for ovarian cancer 3 years earlier and a 2-year spell of unemployment for Mr. T. that had depleted their savings and ended only in the past year. Mrs. T. admitted that Brenda looked like her father's side of the family, from whom Mrs. T. was estranged. She often blamed her husband for Brenda's behavior, and this was the focus of conflict between them. Brenda's answers to questions about her life revealed sleep disturbance, weight loss, difficulty concentrating at school, and a lack of pleasure in ballet and theater. The therapist referred her for a medication consultation, and she was placed on a serotonin reuptake inhibitor. This resolved her depressive symptoms, and her behavior began to improve after the therapist coached her parents in more productive ways of dealing with her. The therapist also attempted to deal with the interlocking triangle with Mr. T.'s extended family, but Mrs. T. was unwilling to touch it.

An example of the problem being exclusively in the child was the frightening case of Irene W., 8 years old. Irene's mother was a single woman living in public housing. She brought Irene to therapy at the urging of the school psychologist, who thought Irene's sudden deterioration in her school work might be due to conflicts with her mother. Her mother appeared worried and harried, but she seemed caring with Irene. In taking the genogram, the therapist discovered plenty of stress that could account for behavioral problems in a child: the mother's job and money worries and a father who had been killed in a drug deal gone sour about a year previously, to name the two biggest. As Irene was leaving with her mother at the end of the session, the therapist noticed that Irene was dragging her foot. Her mother said that this dragging had begun about 3 months earlier and was getting worse. The therapist referred Irene to the pediatrics clinic at the local hospital, which in turn referred her to a tertiary-care hospital. There physicians discovered that Irene had a nonmalignant brain tumor that they removed surgically.

Another way for a potential triangle to become activated is for a third person, sensitized to the conflict in a particular dyad, to move into the role of peacemaker or supporter for the one perceived to be the victim. One 45-year-old woman who was trying to make peace between her husband and her brother-in-law (who was her husband's business partner) described how she had regularly interceded with her parents for her younger sister when they were children. We will offer more in the next chapter on the mechanisms of triangle activation. It's useful to keep in mind that, whatever the mechanisms of activation, we should always think of relationship triangles as structure, movement, process, and functions.

The *structure* of a relationship triangle concerns the spatial representation of the closeness and distance influenced by the conflict that exists in the relationship space between three people. Within that relationship space, there is a constant flow of emotional energy and communication, verbal and nonverbal. This flow contains varying mixtures of affect—for instance, negative and positive feelings, and varying degrees of emotional intensity invested in those feelings. We call this emotional flow *relationship process.*

The relationship process in a triangle can be calm, in which case the triangle is dormant; or it can be reactive, in which case the triangle is active. Reactive process produces *movement* within the relationship, which drives and changes the structure of the triangle. Movement means people maneuvering toward and away from each other, physically or emotionally ("pursuit" and "distance"). Movement is the result of the underlying emotional process in each individual and within their relationships. Such movement can be spontaneous, as when a man's anxiety increases and he automatically becomes silent, sad, and withdrawn. His partner observes this and, worried, asks him what's wrong. He says, "Nothing," and leaves the room. She's hurt by what she interprets as rejection and telephones a friend in another state. She spends an hour on the phone, which angers her partner, and he comes toward her with criticism about the phone bill.

Not all movement is reactive; we can also plan it—as the result of clinical intervention to uncover emotional process. With the couple described above, their therapist could suggest to the woman that she wait for the man to tell her what's wrong rather than ask him. This should not imply that she is doing anything wrong in expressing her concern. On the contrary. However, his typical response to that concern may be concealing the emotional process that includes his dependence on her (as his reaction to her movement by phone toward her friend suggests). Her ability to manage her worry and refrain from asking what's wrong may produce movement on his part, which shows his dependence more explicitly than a complaint about the phone bill.

Movement has an impact on structure, as people move toward and away from each other. The architecture of the triangle changes in response to movement. Whatever the change of structure, and whatever the level of reactivity in the process, we assume that every triangle serves a *function* for the three people involved and for the relationship system as a whole. Thus, structure, process, movement, the mechanisms of triangle activation, and the function the triangle serves are interwoven and mutually influential.

The family, or any other relationship system, can be viewed structurally as a *network* of potential triangles that interlock with one another. (For instance, the husband and wife in a family are two points with connections to each of their children, various in-laws, friends, and others.) These triangles are dormant when the level of emotional arousal in the individuals and the tension in the relationship are low. Stress triggers emotional arousal within the individuals, thereby increasing the tension in the relationship dyad. The combination of these factors (stress, emotional arousal, and tension) activates the triangle. It produces automatic, reactive movement within the triangular structure and modifies that structure. For instance, one parent talks a lot to his child and ignores his wife. This movement and the resulting structural modification of the triangle operate to contain the tension and maintain the system's equilibrium. It does this sometimes by the formation of symptoms in one individual and sometimes in relationship conflict. Thus, the triangle serves a stabilizing, or homeostatic, function for the system. For example, Jane F. spent much of her time with Jennifer because of concern for her poor socialization at school. Peter felt rejected, but, rather than take up that feeling with Jane, he got upset with Jennifer for her poor school performance. His upset was misdirected, but the triangle gave his upset a stabilizing, dysfunctional outlet into Jennifer.

It's important to note the difference between serving a function and being functional. The homeostatic function of the triangle works *against* what is functional for the system and its individual members. Many people have vigorously challenged the idea that symptomatic behavior is functional—especially the idea that people somehow benefit from their troubles. Haley resolves this issue by saying that symptoms don't really exist to serve a function, but to act as if they do may be useful clinically. We believe that people develop symptoms to feel better, and in that sense symptoms have a function. However, eventually the symptom has the effect of leading to dysfunction in the individual or the system over time.

When the clinician sees a triangle, he or she can think that it's serving one of the following functions: stabilizing an unstable dyad, displacing dyadic conflict, or avoiding intimacy in a dyad. The structure of the triangle can be assumed to have been formed by underlying tension or anxiety. A triangle isn't a deliberate or rational process, but a reactive emotional one. We can observe and test the structure, and the testing will uncover the original reactive emotional process, which we can then deal with.

Triangles have functions, but they aren't functional. Stabilizing unstable dyads, displacing conflict, and avoiding intimacy may be natural responses to anxiety, but they militate against what we assume is functional: autonomous individuals who are in one-on-one personal relationships. Triangles become activated in a given emotional system consistently over time, and they work against the possibility of individual autonomy and personal relationships. Ultimately, that is the real reason dealing with them in therapy is so important.

Jeff and Annemarie Y. were a couple married for 6 months before presenting themselves for treatment. Jeff was a 21-year-old police officer who also worked as a carpenter. Annemarie was a 25-year-old bank teller. Both of them felt trapped in a suffocating marriage, forcing them to do things they didn't want to do and become the kind of people they didn't want to be. Jeff was a workaholic, unfaithful, and resentful; Annemarie was critical, hurt, and angry.

The pair had known each other since Jeff was in high school, and their relationship had always been tempestuous. They had had a "wonderful" honeymoon in Aruba but began fighting almost immediately upon their return. Annemarie was critical of Jeff's long hours at work, his tendency to give orders, and his refusal to help with housework. Jeff complained that he was tired of the fighting and resented Annemarie's constant criticism. They had overextended themselves financially by buying a house so early (the *stress*), and this especially bothered Jeff. He was anxious and felt inadequate as a provider (the *emotional arousal*). He dealt with his upset by working even longer hours (*movement* away from Annemarie), which produced more criticism from her (the *tension* in the dyad). With these factors in place, Jeff began to respond more affirmatively to the warmth and flirtation of Susan, a pretty civilian aide at the police station. She had been showing Jeff her attraction to him for months by kidding, engaging him in conversation at change of shift, and telling him risqué jokes. Jeff had enjoyed the flirtation but had avoided any positive action. Finally he asked Susan to have a drink after work. One drink became two, and they ended up in bed in her apartment. Thus Jeff's moves toward Susan activated an extramarital affair triangle, with Jeff and Susan on the inside and Annemarie on the outside (the triangle's *structure*).

If Annemarie hadn't discovered it, the affair might have temporarily stabilized this rocky new marriage (the triangle's *function*). Someone (Annemarie refused to say who, but Jeff suspects it was Susan's previous lover) called Annemarie and told her about Jeff and Susan. Annemarie promptly called Jeff's parents, who took Annemarie's side and joined her in criticism of and pressure on Jeff (an *interlocking triangle*). This move unearthed an interesting piece of *process* about the affair triangle: Jeff claimed to be unaffected by his parents' reaction to the affair because "They've always blamed me for everything; they never defend me." He said that Annemarie's criticism was just a duplication of what he'd always gotten from his parents. Susan's warmth and admiration were a welcome relief from that criticism, and Jeff was unwilling to give her up. There was a paradigm for this nuclear family triangle in Jeff's extended family. The two triangles interlocked when activated by Jeff's affair. A dysfunctional affair triangle, designed to stabilize the marriage, thus resulted in chaos.

In the remainder of this chapter, we focus on structure—defining it, describing the various kinds of structure you will see in triangles, and specifying the implications of triangular structure for clinical work. We deal with process and function in Chapters 5 and 6.

DISSECTING A TRIANGLE'S STRUCTURE

The structure of a triangle is the three people in it and the relationship space between them. The relationship space includes such things as closeness and distance, the emotional climate, and the degree of tension and anxiety among the three and between each person in the three pairs. When most people think of a relationship triangle, the model that occurs to them is three lines on a piece of paper. This is okay, but there is a flaw in thinking of relationship triangles that way: A geometric triangle is too static and lacks the fluidity and the possibility of movement present in relationship triangles. To explain a triangle's structure as both constraining and fluid, we have already suggested the image of a rubber band. The three people stay together, but their freedom of movement is circumscribed by the need to move in response to each other to keep the rubber band from falling. In this situation, a change in the position of one will necessarily create a change in the position of the others or an increased tension between them. The rubber band will keep the sum of the distances among the three people at a constant figure. If one moves away, the other two will pull closer to each other.

People can experience closeness or distance between them as emotionally positive or negative. Closeness and distance refer to the intensity of attachment and the amount of involvement between people, and, sometimes, the degree of their physical proximity. Closeness doesn't necessarily mean affection, nor does distance necessarily mean animosity. Sometimes people feel loved and cared for in a close relationship; sometimes they feel smothered. The closeness between a mother and daughter is sometimes quite enjoyable for them. They go shopping together, they talk things over with one another, they see each other as best friends. But sometimes their closeness turns sour—one or the other feels crowded, controlled, trapped. They fight, criticize, explode in anger and tears. The usual result is reactive distance. The same variability is true about distance. Sometimes people feel relief, freedom, and respect in a distant relationship. Sometimes they feel uncared for, ignored, alone. A therapist working with triangles does well not to assume anything about people's experience about the emotional double-sidedness of closeness and distance, but asks.

Closeness and distance are relative terms defined by past experiences and by how much comfort people have experienced in specific relationships. People search for that mixture of closeness and distance in which the tug of caring and being cared about can be experienced as satisfactory, but they can maintain the ability to remain individuals not fused with another without discomfort. Unfortunately, in relationship systems, this amount of space between self and other will vary among members of the system, with circumstances, and from time to time. There is no "right" amount of space between people. If it works for the people involved, then it's "right." Twosomes have to struggle to get close to this "right," comfortable position with both willing to compromise to get there.

Quite apart from how people feel about the closeness or distance between themselves and others, we should make another distinction between kinds of closeness and distance. Closeness can be a kind of *functional attachment*. This allows people in a relationship to preserve their boundaries and their autonomy in thinking, feeling, and action while they remain connected in a personal way to each other. Alternatively, closeness can be reactive and driven by anxiety, a kind of dependent clinging or *anxious attachment* that says, implicitly or explicitly, "Please don't leave me; I'll do anything to keep you. If you leave, something terrible will happen." Similarly, distance can be a deliberate and planned exercise to deal appropriately with a developmental or relationship problem. It can also be a reactive response to avoid a problem that should be dealt with.

It's worthwhile noting here that the reactive feelings aren't the problem; they're simply a fact. People feel what they feel. We're all reactive at the feeling level; anything else would make us robots. The problem is what we do with those reactive feelings—how we manage them. Anger acted out is often destructive. Anger managed by talking about it and the underlying hurt is useful.

Anxious attachment is the sort of attachment filled with reactive emotion that controls people's behavior in relationships. A pursuer who is anxiously attached to someone may cling to that person in response to anxiety about abandonment; a distancer who is anxiously attached may withdraw as a response to anxiety about rejection or being controlled. Both are reactive behaviors driven by anxiety, and neither are examples of emotional maturity. Both illustrate the flip sides of anxious attachment.

Betty and Jim O. came to therapy complaining of marital conflict. Jim was hurt and angry about Betty's emotional coldness and distance from him; Betty was fed up with Jim's irresponsible approach to life. In taking the history and genogram, the therapist learned that Betty had been in individual therapy for a long time because of her difficulty in dealing with her extended family. She had always taken responsibility for her parents and siblings, but they had never appreciated her and constantly criticized her for not doing enough, especially her mother. Betty reported great satisfaction with individual therapy, because her therapist had told her that the only solution to her mother's impossible behavior was to stay away from her. She had felt "wonderful" ever since. A little less than a year before Betty and Jim had come to marriage therapy, Betty's father, with whom she had always had a better relationship, died. Betty didn't go to the funeral because she didn't want to see her mother. She believed that she had solved her problem with her mother; now she wanted to move on to the issue of her marriage.

A therapist used to thinking about triangles would see that Betty had been caught all her life in her primary parental triangle. Exploring its particulars, the therapist found that Betty and her mother had always had a reactively distant and critical relationship, and what parental comfort and praise she received, she received from her father. Betty reported that she had avoided her mother, but had taken some of the responsibility for the other children to lessen her mother's criticism. Her father had owned a bar and wasn't around much, so Betty spent a lot of time by herself and avoided showing anyone any of her vulnerability or softness.

Her marriage to Jim had activated a new triangle, the in-law triangle. Her parents (more specifically her mother) were at one point, she was at another, and Jim was at the third. Betty's defensive distancing and coldness turned out to be the way she handled upset with Jim

whenever she felt demands or criticism coming from him. That duplicated the way she had handled demands and criticism from her
mother. The advantage of thinking about that dynamic as a triangle
makes it crystal clear that *continuing to distance from her mother only reinforces the marital problem.* Instead, the therapist worked long, hard,
and gently with Betty to experiment with ways of handling her reactions to her mother while maintaining a connection to her.

The other side of the marital problem was Jim's demands for
more open affection and demonstrativeness from Betty, and his criticism of her when she couldn't give it to him. Jim made the connection
with another in-law triangle: His parents and only brother had died in
a fire in their home when he was in college. He told the therapist that
his attitude toward Betty, who was already his girlfriend at that time,
had changed immediately. He had become much more emotionally
needy, and she had responded with warmth and generous comfort-
ing. He accused her of changing after they started to live together,
and now he was often openly critical. Looking at this dynamic as a triangle forced the therapist to think about how Jim could get some of
his emotional needs met without depending entirely on Betty. When
the person or persons at the third point of a triangle are dead, or otherwise unavailable, it can be useful to send a patient to other people
who were connected to absent family members. Jim admitted he had
had little if anything to do with his relatives on either side after his
parents' and brother's funeral. The therapist worked with him as he
experimented with making contact with those relatives and forming
relationships with some of them.

Aspects of Triangular Structure

Four aspects of triangle structure are useful for clinical work. They
are (1) the fixedness and fluidity of the triangle, (2) each individual's
position in the triangle, (3) the location of pain and discomfort in the
triangle, and (4) the distribution of symptoms in the triangle.

Fixedness and Fluidity of Triangles

Fixedness and fluidity concern how much rigidity is in the structure
of a triangle. Three people whose relationships with one another are
not driven by reactive emotion constitute a potential, or dormant triangle. A couple and their son disagree about how much of an allowance he needs at college. The couple argue about it, each hears the

other person's position, and they decide. They present their decision to their son, he argues with them, and perhaps presents a reasonable point that his parents had not thought about. They modify their decision and resolve the issue.

By contrast, three people whose connections with one another are driven by reactive emotion are in an active triangle. An active triangle's structure can vary from being somewhat fluid, capable of changing its structural form, to being rigidly fixed. An active triangle is *fluid* to the extent that the degree of closeness and distance among the persons changes over time. Some fixity is present, but reactive movement takes place, and positions shift within a more or less narrow range. The couple and their son are trying to come to agreement about the son's college allowance, but cannot. Sometimes mother and son are allies against the father, who they believe is being unreasonable about the money. Sometimes father and son try to work it out, but the mother keeps butting in, so father and son turn against her. At still other times, father and mother agree that the son's expenses are excessively high, and they agree that they need to rein him in. The alliances keep shifting, the movement is constant, but reactive emotion drives everything, and issues are never really settled.

A triangle is *fixed* to the extent that the closeness or distance in each twosome stays the same with relatively little movement. Although even in fixed triangles some structural changes occur occasionally, the change is within a very narrow range. Under stress, highly fixed triangles usually return to their characteristic structure. The viewpoints, positions, and movement of individuals in triangles are more predictable the more fixed the triangle. Again, the couple and their son are trying to decide son's allowance, but cannot. Here, however, the parents are rigidly together and unyielding, refusing even to listen to the points their son is raising. The son becomes depressed out of his frustration at trying to deal with them.

The symptomatic expression of triangle activation usually takes the form of relationship conflict (or a cutoff in extreme cases) and/ or dysfunction in an individual (such as anxiety, depression, or physical illness). Clinical experience suggests that the more fixed a triangle's structure, the more malignant its effects. Overt conflicts that shift around from relationship to relationship usually characterize a relatively fluid triangle. Individual symptoms that move around the system may also characterize fluid triangles, with each person taking his or her turn at having symptoms. Nevertheless, when the family presents with symptoms firmly settled in one person, usually the triangle is stubbornly fixed. This in turn stabilizes the location of the symptoms in one person. For example, in the family of someone with a chronic illness such as schizophrenia, rheumatoid arthritis, ulcerative colitis, or end-stage renal disease, the triangles get organized around the chronic illness. They often become fixed, to the point of total rigidity and immovability. In systems terms, this makes it more difficult for the person with the symptoms to give up the patient role. Usually, the more functional a given emotional system, the more fluid the triangles produced in that system. The less functional the emotional system, the more fixed are the triangles produced.

For example, Alex and Joan W., both 48, and their 22-year-old daughter, Julie, were fighting all the time about Julie's lack of success at Oberlin and the unsuitability of her musician boyfriends. (They identified the problem as in Julie.) Joan got worried and she began to bombard Julie with instruction and advice. Julie started to fight with her mother and took to asking her father for money to go out for the evening, thus avoiding Joan. (At that point the problem had moved and was seen as in the mother.) When Alex responded positively to Julie, Joan moved in with outrage toward Alex, and in turn he distanced from Joan's anger into the refuge of his study. (They now saw the problem as in the marriage.) When later Julie left to go back to Oberlin, Alex and Joan took a vacation together where they had time to close ranks in worrying about their darling daughter. (The perception of the problem had moved again, this time back to being in Julie.) In this triangle, constant movement was taking place, and everyone was uncomfortable at various times. Joan sometimes cried and sometimes screamed over her anxiety about Julie; Alex frequently felt badgered by Joan and placed in the middle by Julie; and Julie felt criticized and unappreciated. This triangle was full of reactive process that drove shifting movement and changed its structure. Nevertheless, its relative fluidity predicts that this family will get more benefit from clinical intervention than might otherwise be the case.

An example of a triangle more fixed in its movement is the case of Grace V. Grace was a seriously depressed 50-year-old woman repeatedly hospitalized after making threats to drive her car into an abutment. She had been married for 25 years, and over that time, her husband, Bill, and her mother, Harriet, had become good friends. Grace felt criticized and misunderstood by them, while they felt hopeless and angry about her depression and her "manipulation" of the family. Grace and Bill were sometimes allies against Harriet's interference, and sometimes Grace and Harriet could have a calm and mutually supportive conversation. Most of the time, however, Grace found herself in the outside position. She was the butt of her mother's and her husband's "helpful" and "constructive" criticism and was unable to make a positive connection with either of them. The fixity of this triangle increased Grace's frustration, her feeling of being trapped, and her sense of a lack of control in her life. Her depressive symptoms got worse and worse, and she developed life-threatening asthma attacks, which also caused repeated hospitalizations. Although her psychiatric and medical illnesses went in cycles, even at the best point in the cycles, Grace was consistently the designated symptom bearer.

A potential triangle is exemplified by a mother, father, and son who can usually relate one-on-one with each other. (A mother and father can have their own relationship time without their son; the mother and her son can show affection without the father becoming resentful, and the father and his son can discuss the son's report card without the mother stepping in to "protect" her son.) It is only under some degree of stress (the son fails sophomore year math) that the potential triangle becomes an active, though still fluid, triangle. Once the triangle is active, reactive movement begins: Because the father gets anxious about his son's math grade, he automatically (i.e., without thinking about it) starts to criticize his son and then moves into the distant position by saying he has some errands to do and leaving the house. The son turns to his mother for protection by saying the grade wasn't his fault, and the mother reassures her son and promises to speak to the father. After a time, the father reacts to being on the outside by speaking to his wife about his concern for their son. At that point, the parents present a united front by deciding to ground their son for 2 weeks. This puts the son on the outside as the object of their concern. As the stress level subsides, one could predict that this fluid triangle would return (temporarily) to being a potential triangle.

An affair is usually part of a rigidly structured triangle, where the unfaithful spouse and the lover are overly close, and the betrayed spouse is in the outside position. The structure of such a triangle almost never changes, at least as far as the relationship between the betrayed spouse and the lover is concerned. Even here, however, there is some fluidity: The relationships between the unfaithful spouse and the lover and between the two spouses fluctuate over time. The affair breaks up, and the spouses temporarily reconcile. This is followed by increased distance between the spouses and the reactivation of the affair.

Affairs are sometimes "triangles of revolution," which usually become quite fixed. A triangle of revolution is one in which one member of a twosome is locked in and constrained by the dynamics of the relationship into an adaptive position. We have used the term "adaptive" for some time.[2] The adaptive position is one in which, like a chameleon, we give up our own agenda and beliefs to knuckle under to the agenda and beliefs of the other. Like the chameleon, we do it to survive, but the price we pay is the surrender of self—the production of a no-self state.

Over time, the adaptive position leads to mild to moderate depression and acting out of anger; that acting out can come as an affair or some similar triangular response. Father Edward F., a Roman Catholic priest who was an assistant pastor in a suburban parish, was sent to therapy by his bishop when someone told the bishop of an affair he was having with a married woman in the parish. Edward, 38 years old, had been in the parish for 3 years when the affair began. From the time he had arrived, the pastor, a much older and more conservative man, had rigidly controlled Edward's activities as assistant pastor, leaving little room for Edward to express his own ideas and creativity as a priest. Edward had become increasingly frustrated and had recently asked for a transfer, but the bishop refused. A few days after the refusal, Arlene G. had come to the rectory for counseling about her marriage. Arlene was a beautiful 35-year-old woman, who admitted she had been attracted to Edward for some time. The attraction became mutual, and they began an affair.

How do dormant triangles become active and fluid, and how do fluid triangles become fixed? One factor is that people repeat certain patterns of relating repeatedly. These patterns become "conditioned responses" that people engage in and respond to in essentially fixed ways. Over time, people believe that they know each other. They make assumptions about each other, and they stop listening because they "know" what the other will say and do. Such assumptions become self-fulfilling prophecies, fixing beliefs and behavior in rigidity. By contrast, if a person realizes that he or she can never really know another person, he listens to that person to get to know him or her as best he can. Faulty assumptions are corrected, and one-on-one relationships are more possible. Triangles become less fixed, and it takes higher levels of stress to push potential triangles to activation.

---

[2] For example, in Guerin et al. (1987, pp. 131–132).

Two other factors that shift triangles from potential to fluid to fixed are the level of stress in the system and the system's premorbid level of functioning. These factors work together. In a relatively functional family, ordinary stress will not move fluid triangles to fixity, but very high stress might very well do so. By contrast, in systems with low levels of differentiation, even ordinary events will be stressful enough to move triangles to fixity or keep them fixed.

The following is an example of a fixed triangle in a relatively functional family—a family under stress because of the death of a key member, complicated by one of the biggest stressors around—a wedding. Grandma G. used to be Aaron G.'s favorite grandparent and he her favorite grandchild. That all changed when his father died, and the conflict between Aaron's mother and Aaron's paternal grandmother came into the open. The immediate trigger for the conflict was the will and the dividing of certain mementos. Aaron found himself disappointed by his grandmother's behavior. He never mentioned his anger to her but became more distant, calling and writing less and less frequently.

Everything seemed okay at family gatherings and special occasions, until Aaron's wedding approached. Grandma G. insisted on inviting some people Aaron's mother didn't like, and all hell broke loose. Aaron and Grandma G. had a terrific fight—their first ever. Aaron was angry that his grandmother was upsetting his mother. Of course, most of the fuel for this triangle was the grief all three people felt for the death of Aaron's father and his absence from the wedding.

Grandma G. had always shown favoritism toward Aaron. Since she and Aaron's mother had never gotten along, when Aaron's father died the conflict between the two women exploded. Aaron was so caught between them that he either distanced from both of them or took his mother's side. His father's funeral had been difficult, not only because people were sad, but because the tension was so great you could almost see it. Aaron had felt it was his job to keep things calm, but he had resented being in that position. He had thought his brothers should take more responsibility for his mother and grandmother, since he didn't know what to do about their disputes. His fiancee felt that everyone was picking on Aaron. She thought he ought to get away from both his mother and Grandma G., and then he would feel better. Thus the triangles began to multiply and interlock.

In this family, whose members typically functioned at a high level, the stress increased the fixity and intensity of the Aaron–Grandma G.–mother triangle around the times of the stressors (the funeral and the wedding). In a higher-functioning family with the same history and stressors, the reactions would be similar but less intense and less fixed. In a lower-functioning family, you can predict that the stressors would have produced far more fixed and intense reactions.

Positions in Triangles

A second clinically important aspect of structure concerns the positions people occupy in the triangle. Structurally individuals may occupy three positions: inside, outside, or caught in the middle. The *inside* is a position occupied by the two participants in the triangle who are joined by (1) emotional closeness (e.g., the oldest daughter's special relationship with her father and how it affects the relationships of both of them with the mother and younger brothers and sisters), (2) a common agenda (e.g., the father and son who use frequent fishing trips to get around the wife and mother's objections to their drinking), or (3) dependent clinging to one another (e.g., the mother and daughter who can't go anywhere or do anything separately in the months after the husband–father's death). The *outside* is the position occupied by the member of the triangle more emotionally distant from the other two. The outsider can be in that position because of being actively excluded from the relationship by the other two (e.g., the 5- and 8-year-old brothers who won't let their 6-year-old sister play with them), or by deliberately distancing him- or herself from the other two (e.g., the man who won't speak to his sister because she is dating someone of another religion). Sometimes the outsider is being ignored, sometimes he or she is distancing by choice. Sometimes, too, the outsider is the one around whom the other two organize, putting pressure on him or her to change (e.g., the man whose wife and mother are trying to get him to stop drinking). The one *caught in the middle* is the member of the triangle who is caught emotionally by the tension in the relationship between the other two and attempts to make peace between the combatants (e.g., the parentified child who, faced with daily combat between his or her parents, attempts futilely to make peace). Sometimes the peacemaking may be carried on explicitly. It may also be done implicitly by dealing with the tension in an unconscious way through acting out and thus drawing the other two together. Each of these structural positions is reinforced and kept in place by the emotional reactivity of each individual and by the stabilizing function of the triangle.

We can also define these structural positions by the degree to which reactivity decides the behavior of the person in the position. Table 4.1 diagrams the matrix in which the three positions and these emotional characteristics can intersect. In the *reactive* positions (nos. 1, 2, and 3 in Table 4.1), the person reacts unthinkingly to the behavior of others. In the *adaptive* positions (nos. 4, 5, and 6), a variant of the reactive, a person gives up one's own program and knuckles under to relationship pressure to behave in a certain way or go along with someone else's program. These six possibilities are by definition dysfunctional and will be found in some combination in all active triangles. In therapy, *experimental* positions (nos. 7, 8, and 9) can be devised as a strategy for individual and relationship change. In therapy, experiments to shift structure and unearth process can be devised. People are urged to move toward a different position (from the insider to the outsider, for example). Simultaneously, they must carefully monitor their own internal emotional process and observe the relationship process. In the *functional* positions (nos. 10, 11, and 12), one is emotionally and physically available to a relationship, open to negotiating differences of opinion, able to take a strong "I-position" when necessary, and willing to allow the other to take the lead in areas where the other is more competent. When at least one member of the triangle is occupying a functional position vis-à-vis the other two, the triangle has been deactivated. The therapist should choose the highest functioning individual in the triangle, probably *not* someone in the adaptive position. The goal is to move him or her through one or more experimental positions to a functional position.

Here is an example of how thinking about positions in triangles can be useful in a clinical situation. Joel and Marcy T. came to therapy complaining about Joel's alcoholic drinking, which he had been unable to stop in spite of joining AA and a 4-week stay in a rehabilita-

TABLE 4.1. Types of Positions in Triangles

	Insider	Outsider	Caught in the middle
Reactive	1	2	3
Adaptive	4	5	6
Experimental	7	8	9
Functional	10	11	12

tion facility. In filling out a genogram, the therapist discovered that Marcy wasn't the only person concerned about Joel's drinking; Joel's mother frequently talked with Marcy about what they should do to get him to stop, and both of them pressured him, together and separately, to change his behavior. Joel went to AA meetings regularly because Marcy and his mother asked him to, and his stay in rehabilitation was the result of an ultimatum from them. Thus, Marcy and her mother-in-law were both in the insider reactive positions, joined in their pressure on Joel, and reacting unthinkingly and emotionally to his drinking. Joel was in the outsider adaptive position (remember that adaptive here means giving up one's own program and knuckling under to the program of others—see p. 65). Joel was equally reactive to his wife and his mother, so that all three were reactive to the drinking or to the feelings aroused by the drinking. Joel was under constant pressure to change to please his wife and mother but never had a position of his own. This case was going nowhere unless this triangle could be modified. Marcy and Joel's mother could try to be more tolerant of Joel's drinking and stop pressuring him about it; Joel could try to stop drinking again. It would be futile, because they were caught in the invisible web of a powerful and sticky triangle. The therapist realized that the positions each person occupied in the triangle relative to each other had to be changed. Marcy and Joel's mother had to work on being less reactive *while separating from each other around the issue of Joel's drinking.* Joel needed to take a stand for himself (rather than being compliant for his wife's and mother's sakes) *while moving toward an insider position with his wife vis-à-vis his mother.*

The therapist met Joel's mother, who had a history of depression and panic disorder. Her high anxiety and incoherent responses in the interview led the therapist to conclude that Marcy was the most functional member of the triangle. He chose, therefore, to work with Marcy to experiment with various moves in the triangle. He suggested that Marcy back off from her focus on Joel's drinking and leave Joel and his mother to battle it out without her. The therapist's plan was to move Marcy away from her insider position with Joel's mother in the triangle. That would include making a clear statement to Joel about where she stands, stopping her fruitless attempts to get him to stop drinking, and maintaining her connection with her mother-in-law without talking about Joel. This would diminish the pressure on Joel enough so that he could deal with his mother one-on-one and could decide what *he* wanted to do about his drinking.

The Distribution of Discomfort in Triangles

A third aspect of structure concerns pain. The distribution of discomfort among the three people in a triangle is variable. It depends on the nature of the twosomes in the triangle and on the operating principles of the three individuals. (We're talking about degrees of discomfort; no one in an active triangle is entirely comfortable.) For example, the outsider isn't always the person with the most heartache. If the outsider is a distancer being ignored by a cozy twosome, he or she is probably comfortable—up to a certain point. A husband is often very happy to have his wife and mother be good friends, especially if it diminishes their demands on him. When or if the twosome becomes conflictual, the outsider is the most comfortable one *if he is a distancer.* He may be working to remain on the outside by resisting any efforts to pull him in. The distancer husband whose wife and mother are quarreling will usually do anything to stay out of their fight.

If the outsider is a pursuer, however, he or she may be uncomfortable in the outsider position and actively try to mediate or solve the relationship conflict between the close twosome. When the two insiders are a cozy twosome and the outsider is a pursuer whom they are ignoring, he or she may be very uncomfortable and move toward one or both of them to "get in."

The discomfort is almost evenly distributed when positions in the triangle are constantly shifting and there is significant relationship reactivity. By contrast, when the structure is fixed over time, where the symptom resides in one person, and where little movement takes place, the discomfort is usually concentrated in one member of the triangle.

Jake S. was a 23-year-old college graduate living at home and working as a carpenter. He was constantly at odds with his father, who was overprotective of him and very critical of him. Jake adored his father and was very hurt by his father's negativity toward him. His responses to the negativity fluctuated between explosive anger and withdrawal into depression, marked at its worst with passive suicidal ideation. Jake's mother was a pursuer who tried to keep the peace between Jake and his father. Both of them turned to her for comfort, reassurance, and an ally. When Jake and his father were not fighting, they were extremely close, doing things together, talking, and "hanging out."

In this triangle, who was feeling worst at any given time would be hard to predict because the alliances and relationships shifted so much. However, if Jake's mother and father were to move into a fixed alliance against Jake, pressuring him to change and otherwise not having much to do with him, it is completely predictable that Jake would quickly become consistently the most uncomfortable member of the triangle. When Jake and his father fight, his mother has always become the most uncomfortable one.

Symptom Location in Triangles

A fourth aspect of structure concerns the location of the symptom. Who has the symptom, and how is that linked to the structural position the symptom bearer occupies? The symptom bearer in a family can occupy any of the structural positions. However, in a triangle where someone is in the outsider, *adaptive* position, that person is the one most likely to develop the symptom. The treatment approach varies depending on the nature of the symptom and on the position occupied by the symptom bearer.

Nathan R. exemplifies a symptom-bearer who was in the caught-in-the-middle position. He is a 38-year-old lawyer who had an affair and now cannot decide between staying with his lover and returning to his wife (the symptom). Nathan got married during law school to Ruth, a woman with whom he had always had an excellent relationship, one with much chemistry and passion. During his dating years he had dated only Italian women, of whom his Jewish mother strongly disapproved. Ruth, however, is Jewish, and someone of whom his mother very much approved. Their excellent relationship continued until Ruth decided she wanted children, a decision much favored by Nathan's mother. When Ruth told Nathan, "We've been married for 7 years; it's time to have kids," Nathan's reply was, "I married you to take care of *me.*"

They had fertility problems, adopted a daughter, and then had a biological son. The adopted child, Lauren, turned out to have learning disabilities, and Ruth's shame and disappointment meant that she could never make a real connection with her. Nathan made an excellent connection with Lauren, and got angry with Ruth because he did not believe she was really trying with Lauren. He felt strongly that Ruth was much more emotionally tied to their son, Luke, and was not a good mother to Lauren. In addition Nathan objected to Ruth's spending patterns, her lack of interest in housework, and her commitment to art as an avocation. So, Nathan had an affair and moved out of his home.

Nathan's affair was with a very sexual Italian Catholic woman with whom he lived for 3 years. When it came time for his divorce from Ruth to be completed, Nathan left his lover and came back home to try to make the marriage work. His lover became depressed and threatened suicide, and Nathan started seeing her and having sex with her again. At this point the lover began to call Ruth and taunt her with Nathan's visits. Nathan told the therapist that he really loved his lover, but what he always wanted was his home and family; he said he felt "caught in the middle." The clinical hypothesis here is that Nathan's symptom of obsessional indecision will resolve if he can call a moratorium on both relationships. He does this by going off and being by himself (thus altering his position in the triangle from reactive, caught-in-the-middle to experimental outsider).

If he does this, he will also be confronted with the inner emotional turmoil, which, up to now, he has been "self-medicating" with his affair. Sorting through this turmoil will take him through several interlocking triangles. These include the triangle with Ruth and his daughter Lauren, the one with Ruth and his mother, and finally his relationship with his mother as a part of his primary parental triangle. All these interlocking triangles have been activated as serial displacements of his individual problems with his mother as he bounced back and forth between rebellion and compliance. During these serial displacements, the core problem is buried under mounds of relationship debris. The shift in the triangular structure, however, surfaces all of this relationship process to where it can be seen and dealt with.

A symptom bearer in the outside position was Roger N., a young executive whose wife, Melissa, had stopped taking contraceptives at Roger's urging and in spite of her own reluctance. Although she had been reluctant, once she had children, she developed something she had never experienced before: an area of competence. She became a child-rearing "expert" and was determined that she would raise her children perfectly. Among other things, this included telling Roger how to relate to their children, and Roger was having none of that. This created the conflict that brought them to therapy, and Roger's "symptom" was his inability to allow his wife to have this one area of competence and leadership. He rejected out of hand any suggestion she made about how he might deal with the children.

He described himself as having substantial trouble with authority—"*no one* tells me what to do." His problem with authority was tied to his mother's domination of his father. Roger was insistent that his wife would never "have my balls in a jar on the shelf the way my mother had my father's." Roger's symptom was triggered by his out-side position in the triangle with Melissa and their children. The clini-cal hypothesis here is that Roger needs to be able to have a relation-ship with his children without a control struggle with his wife. One way of accomplishing that is to focus on his negative reactivity to be-ing in the outside position and tie it to the interlocking triangle with his parents. The goal would be to move him from the reactive outside position to a functional outside position. From there he could move easily to an inside position with his wife or, at other times, to an inside position with his children. In other words, Roger would have the op-tion of moving in or out at will depending on the context, instead of having only one predictable response to these kinds of situations.

An example of a symptom bearer in the inside position was Eric M. Eric was a 13-year-old boy whom his mother brought to therapy with the symptom of being unable to get up and get to school in the morning. Eric's parents were divorced, and his maternal grandfather and maternal uncle had both died within the last 9 months. During that same period, his father left the New York area for California with Eric's stepmother and stepsiblings. In addition, Eric's mother had been having a love affair with a divorced man, and it had appeared that they would get married. However, the man left and returned to his ex-wife. The losses, especially of male figures, were huge for both Eric and his mother. As a result, Eric became even more emotionally tied to his mother than he had been. The clinical hypothesis is that loosening this tie and freeing Eric up would allow his symptom to dis-appear.

As the clinician intervenes to change the structure of triangles, he or she should carefully track the changes that occur in response to the therapist's interventions and suggested experiments. One way of doing this is to visualize the triangles according to the forms they take. Tracking the triangle's form enables the therapist to get a visual image of the triangle's structure and to follow its movement over time. Tracking also allows the therapist to develop further strategies with movement that will elaborate the process and continue to re-structure the triangle. Visualizing the form of the triangle, and follow-ing the movement within it, provide a road map to track movement and a focus for observation during each visit with the family. The therapist can use this map to direct change in the positions within the triangle and in what is happening inside its borders.

It may be of value for the therapist to draw a picture of the triangle in his or her notes. To do this, look for one prominent, central issue that the family brings to therapy and for what the consistent, predictable positions of the family members are around that issue. Who sides with whom? Who is in the solo position? Who moves toward whom and who moves away from whom? Who are the good guys and who are the bad guys? For example, a child and his or her parents may line up with another child who is distant and isolated in the "bad" position; or a child may end up in the position of being close to both parents who are distant from each other and communicate only through the child.

In the first case, as the situation changes, the daughter and her brother may develop their own relationship, and the distance narrows. The same process occurs between the parents and their son. Then the over closeness begins to disappear between the parents and their daughter. In the second instance, as the process changes, the child stops being the funnel for communications between the parents and develops a one-on-one relationship with each parent that has nothing to do with the other parent. Then the parents begin to talk with each other.

Watching the old film *The Subject Was Roses* provides a good opportunity to practice this kind of tracking. In this movie, a young man has just returned to his parents' apartment in the Bronx from service in World War II. The setting is not dissimilar from that of the more recent *A Bronx Tale*. The story makes it obvious that mother and son have always been close, too close in fact, with the father in a distant and angry outside position. The movie is about the son's first few days at home, and about where his loyalties will lie now that he is "a man." The son's drinking, his war experiences, and his attachment to the family's summer cottage all pull him toward his father. His mother's pain and his old anger at his father as the cause of that pain pull him toward his mother. The parents' distance from each other, the father's miserly control of the money, and the mother's sexual withholding prevent the few moments of tenderness between the spouses from staying one-on-one. As the movie unfolds, we see the son moving back and forth between father and mother. We see his attempt to break free and start his own life. In the final scene, we see how caught the son is in the triangle with his parents, and how the power of their problems with each other keeps him caught.

Although structure is the most easily seen element of a triangle, it is not the only one. We turn now to a consideration of process, movement, and function.

CHAPTER FIVE

Emotional Process within Triangular Structure

SEEING RELATIONSHIP PROCESS

One way of linking the ideas of emotional process and triangles is to see emotional process as internal to the individual. Internal emotional process generates movement toward and away from other people, and movement creates positions vis-à-vis one another. These positions define an interpersonal structure that it is clinically useful to break down into triangles. For example, a fifth-grader fails math. The child and his parents all experience internal emotional arousal of various kinds in response to this stressor. They begin to move around the system as a way of dealing with the discomfort of their emotional arousal: For example, the child feels ashamed and depressed, and withdraws from his parents. His father feels anxious and angry with the child and pursues him with criticism and punishment. The mother feels concerned about the child for failing math, and angry with her husband for his negativity and criticism, which is usually directed at her. She moves toward her husband with her anger and defensiveness about the child. We now have a triangle in which marital conflict has erupted with the focus on the child, who is in the outside position.

This model has plenty of advantages. It's simple and easy to understand. Straightforward interventions follow from it, and they usually provide rapid symptom relief. For example, a therapist might intervene by modifying the triangle's structure: getting people to change experimentally the direction of their movement, and observing and dealing with the behavioral and emotional shifts that occur.

Alternatively, one could work on the internal emotional state of one or more of the individuals involved. The goal is freeing up that individual to move more functionally in the interpersonal system. For example, the therapist might concentrate on the father's disappointment in his son and explore with him his feelings about his own failures in life and about his need to have his child succeed. Or the therapist could concentrate on the child and have him tested for learning disabilities or behavior problems; perhaps he could see him in therapy or send him to a tutor. A third possibility is for the therapist to explore the mother's reaction to anger and her identification with her son. Any of these methods might alter the *triangular* process in the relationship. If it does, it will be successful. If it doesn't, it won't.

However, seeing emotional process as purely intrapersonal has several disadvantages. For one thing, it leaves no room for the interpersonal transmission of anxiety and of other kinds of emotional arousal. It ignores the ability of one person to pick up on another's emotional state and respond to it without any behavioral signals from the first person to the second. In other words, it leaves out the notion of interpersonal relationship process. It doesn't come to grips with the fact that there is process going on *in the relationship space between people.* This emotional process between people is as real as the emotional process within them.

Of course, both notions—internal emotional process and interpersonal relationship process—are abstractions, not directly observable phenomena. Internal emotional process as an abstraction has a long history and is a lot easier to talk about because an entire language has developed in psychology to describe it. Words like repression, anxiety, anger, and self-esteem are so widely used and understood that we take the notion of internal emotional process for granted. Our problem is finding a way to define and talk about what goes on between and among people. We need to go beyond a psychology of the individual to develop a two-person psychology, and even beyond that to develop a psychology of triangles (a three-person psychology) that can account for the interplay of different minds, each with its own agenda. Then we need to find ways of intervening with and operating on that process.

Lonnie and Calvin Z. were working in marital therapy on the lack of emotional and sexual desire Lonnie had been feeling for Calvin.

The therapist had determined that Lonnie had begun losing her feelings for Calvin around the same time a surgeon diagnosed her father with lung cancer. He had since died, and this was difficult for both of them, since her father had been a favorite of both.

The therapist identified several triangles that involved both Lonnie and Calvin, and determined that the triangle with Calvin's mother was putting considerable pressure on the couple. The pressure was particularly intense whenever they returned to their families' homes in Kansas. While there, Lonnie hated going to see Calvin's mother. Lately she had been refusing to accompany Calvin and their two little boys to grandmother's house for an afternoon visit. She begged off, saying her own widowed mother needed her, when what she really thought was that Calvin's mother was an idiot.

The therapist also learned that Calvin had a ritualized relationship with his mother; he made the obligatory, biweekly phone calls, sent cards and letters on Christmas, Mother's Day, and her birthday, and visited several times a year. But the fact was that he disliked his mother. She had been cruel to him as a child, she treated his children coldly, and he couldn't have a personal conversation with her. By the time they were in therapy, however, Calvin focused more on Lonnie's behavior toward his mother than on his own.

The therapist decided to work on the Lonnie–Calvin–Calvin's mother triangle first. Step one was to help Lonnie change her position in the triangle. Lonnie needed to get into an emotionally neutral position with her mother-in-law. The therapist talked to Lonnie about her being a role model for her sons in how you treat in-laws and about the necessity for anyone to have a civil relationship with a partner's mother and their children's grandmother. As Lonnie worked on this and got more neutral about Calvin's mother, the shift in her feelings gave her the chance to think about her feelings about returning to her family home without her father being there and about how she was coping with her mother's grief.

Step two was shifting Calvin's position. The therapist asked Calvin, "As you watch Lonnie working on her relationship with your mother, how much do you think her anger is yours rather than her own?" Calvin answered, "As Lonnie is getting less angry with my mother, I'm getting more angry with her." As the discussion continued, the therapist connected Calvin's anger and the way he behaved toward his mother. Calvin saw how much he needed his mother to be less possessive of him and less controlling of his life. He realized how much his ritualized connection with his mother and the emotional distance between them was a by-product of his mother's intensity and his own anger. The therapist then coached Calvin to narrow the distance between him and his mother by beginning brief, unpredictable how-are-you-doing phone calls, during which he should work on keeping his reactivity down and make certain to share one or two personal pieces of information about himself. The therapist successfully made the connection between Calvin's worry and reactivity about his own parenting and getting his relationship with his mother less tense and more natural. Calvin's motivation to do this work increased because of his own desire to be a good parent and his worry that he might not be.

On their next trip to Kansas, Lonnie and Calvin had changed some patterns. Lonnie went graciously to her in-laws' house. Calvin had been calling his mother several unexpected times. She had really enjoyed the calls and was nicer than usual when they came by to visit. Lonnie thought Calvin was taking more responsibility for his mother, which warmed her to him. Calvin noticed that Lonnie was much sadder about her Dad on this visit, but she spoke about him more than she had been.

Lonnie's lack of sexual desire (an individual symptom) could only be understood in the context of the marriage. That's obvious. What is less obvious is that Lonnie's symptom and Lonnie and Calvin's marital tension were tied to several triangles, and addressing those triangles was an essential part of resolving Lonnie's symptom and the marital tension.

Eighteen months after Lonnie and Calvin had terminated therapy with significant improvement in their sexual relationship, Lonnie returned for a few sessions complaining of "sexual apathy." On exploration, the therapist learned that Lonnie's apathy was apparent outside the bedroom as well as in it. Besides, Lonnie had moved into her father's position as the family's problem-solver. Lonnie's niece, with whom she was close, and Calvin's brother had both been having severe problems in their marriages. Concerned family members were calling Lonnie for advice. Lonnie felt very worried about these relatives and upset with herself because she couldn't fix the trouble. As a result, she began to shut down internally. She was unaware, until she spoke with the therapist, that she was caught again in extended family triangles. That recognition was all she needed at this point to turn things around. Her apathy receded as she began the process of detriangling from these extended family situations.

Defining Interpersonal Emotional Process

The notion of interpersonal relationship process is tied to the old idea of fusion. Fusion concerns internal emotional process as that process relates to an individual's need for autonomy and connection. The activation of a connection with another person creates an emotional conduit between them. Within that conduit *each person's* internal emotional state can play itself out between them and affect what goes on inside each of them. This joining and interaction of the internal emotional process of two (or more) persons in the relationship space between them constitute an emergent reality that we call the *interpersonal relationship process.*

Ways of Talking about Interpersonal Emotional Process

There are several component parts of interpersonal relationship process. They include:

1. *Individual states of emotional arousal.* At any given moment, people may be feeling anxious or confident, depressed or happy, optimistic or pessimistic. They may feel hurt and angry, warm and grateful, distant or close. These feelings may be more or less intense when compared with another time. People may feel more or less vulnerable at any given moment. Furthermore, two or more people who are connected to one another may at any given moment be in the same *or a different* emotional state from one another.

2. *Individual differences in people's ability to control their emotional arousal.* Their emotional states dominate some people, while others can manage them. The behavior of some people is reactive. If you know someone who rarely seems to hear what you're trying to say because he or she flares up with criticism or advice about one small particular, then you know how irritating dealing with emotionally reactive people can be. Their behavior flows directly from their emotional state, with little ability on their part to reflect on their emotional state. They can't choose a course of action based on any other consideration than their emotions. They react as if by reflex, and they have few options or choices about how to manage their feelings. Other people are more reflective. Because they can more competently manage their emotional states, they can choose a course of action for themselves rather than being run by their emotions. They

have options about how to manage their feelings. Ego strength is the capacity for delay.

3. *Variations in the level of attachment in, and the importance of, the specific relationship.* The parent–child relationship in a family, for example, is a lot more intense than the customer–clerk relationship in a delicatessen (depending, of course, on how hungry you are and how long the line). There will usually be intense interpersonal relationship process between family members, while there may or may not be between customer and clerk.

4. *Individual differences in sensitivities to certain forms of behavior or of feelings.* Some people are so sensitized to anger, for instance, that they see it everywhere—even in complete strangers—and react to it intensely. The young server whom you ask for ice in your water responds as if you've asked her to impale herself on your steak knife. Other people are too sensitive to sadness or depression. A child who calls home from college and says to her father, "Are you okay? You sound sad," when in fact her father is fine, is probably overly sensitive to him or to sadness and depression. At the other extreme, some people may be so tuned out that they neglect to pick up emotional signals, even quite strong ones, and even from close family members. One woman told a story of her daughter coming in from a date and running upstairs to her room, tears streaming down her face. The woman and her husband were watching television, and the woman said to her husband, "Gee, I wonder what happened?" Her husband's reply: "Charles Bronson just shot one of the bad guys."

Intervention with Interpersonal Process

The possibility of operating on interpersonal relationship process follows from the idea of differentiation. If you're anxious and I'm not, and if I don't get caught up in your anxiety, I'll neutralize it. You'll begin to feel less anxious. A familiar example from everyday life is the homeowner who notices water dripping from his ceiling. Worried sick, he calls a plumber and, even on the phone, exudes anxiety. "What do you think it is? Can it be fixed? Are we going to have to rebuild the whole bathroom?" The plumber, who's seen it all, stays calm and says he'll be right over. He arrives, finds the problem, and fixes it, all the while acting as if this kind of thing happens a hundred times a day. The homeowner's anxiety decreases as the plumber proceeds, and soon he is chatting with the plumber as if he knew all along it would be no big deal. When the plumber completes the patch job, he mentions the need for more extensive background work to improve the functioning of the bathroom and prevent further leaks. Bowen's belief about the essence of marital therapy also illustrates this point. He said that if a therapist could maintain an emotional connection with both spouses while not getting caught up in the emotional state of either one, or in the relationship process between them, the marriage would get better. Then the couple might (or might not) be open to doing some extended family work to consolidate their gains.

PROCESS QUESTIONS

The *American Heritage Dictionary of the English Language,* third edition, defines process as a series of actions, changes, or functions bringing about a result: for example, the process of digestion; the process of obtaining a driver's license. In that sense, all psychotherapists ask process questions. Yet the nature of their questions flows directly from the model of behavior and therapy that they use. If you watch videotapes of Murray Bowen working, you'll notice that he asks a thousand and one generic questions that he designs to neutralize overflowing affect and anxiety, galvanize the cognitive centers of the brain, and encourage patients to find their own solutions: for example, "How in the world do you figure you get so angry when your mother does that?" Similarly, Aaron Beck's questions in psychotherapy are directed at documenting the connection between a patient's symptom and his or her cognitive distortions and at helping the patient find a way to correct those distortions: "When someone is late coming home, does your mind tend to choose the more dire of two possible explanations?" An analyst asks questions aimed at fostering the transference. Patient: "What are you thinking?" Analyst: "Thinking?"

Our model of questioning borrows the process question from Bowen's formula, but directs questioning more specifically to patterns of cognition, relationship movement, the expression of affect, and triangulation. Like the plumber, we believe in responding to and finding a remedy for the symptom and coming back another day to do the important background work. We leave this return work to the interest and motivation of the patient or family, knowing that they may never pick up on it.

Clinicians working with triangles are interested in the actions, changes, and functions going on inside person *A,* inside person *B,* inside person *C*, between *A* and *B*, between *A* and *C*, and between *B* and *C*. Questions aimed at eliciting those pieces of information are what we're calling *process questions.* "If you have a problem with your son, how does your husband deal with it?" "When your son breaks curfew, what goes on inside you?" These kinds of process questions fulfill several functions: (1) they make implicit emotional process explicit for both the therapist and patients; (2) they place behavior, especially symptomatic behavior, in an interpersonal context; (3) they are the most important way the therapist stays out of triangles with patients.

Sam and Jeannine L. came for treatment after many years of reactive distance and several unsuccessful attempts at marital therapy. In the engagement phase of the therapy, Jeannine for the first time became interested in looking at herself as a part of the problem. Her own hair-trigger emotionality, her preoccupation with her children, and her indifference toward sexual intimacy with her husband became clearer to her.

When Jeannine experimented with initiating sex for the first time in more than 10 years, Sam turned her down—he was "too tired." The therapist saw each of them separately, as part of the normal evaluation phase of therapy. In his session, Sam revealed a long-term affair with Sarah, an operating-room nurse at the hospital where Sam was a highly respected surgeon. He and the therapist discussed the difficulties inherent in this arrangement for both relationships. On the following day Sam began to talk with Sarah about ending the sexual part of their affair.

Sarah responded by calling and telling Jeannine about her relationship with Sam, including some sexual details. The call to Jeannine came on a Sunday morning. The next day Sam and Jeannine were in the therapist's office to deal with the fallout, which was considerable.

The structure of the extramarital affair triangle had been fixed for years with Jeannine in the outside position. The therapist had stirred up the process in Sam, in Jeannine, and in their relationship. In doing so, he had modified the movement in the triangle so that its structure had shifted dramatically, putting Sarah in the outside position. In calling Jeannine, Sarah had made a dramatic and desperate move. She wanted to reestablish the triangle's old structure with her on the inside and Jeannine on the outside. If that couldn't be done, she wanted at least to retaliate for her loss.

To understand better the process in this long-term extramarital affair triangle, let us track the emotional process that fed into it from the beginning of Sam and Jeannine's relationship.

They had met in college. Sam was the only child of immigrant parents from Italy. Both parents, but especially his mother, had an intense emotional attachment to Sam. Going away to college was a chance for Sam to escape their smothering love.

Jeannine was also part of a very intense primary parental triangle, as the special child of her father and of his side of the family. Jeannine's brother was her mother's special child, but her mother was the real outsider in the family: she was from the Pacific Northwest and had almost no contact with her side of the family. Jeannine had felt a lot of pressure from her father's extraordinarily powerful attachment to her. While growing up, she, like Sam, had seen college as a liberating opportunity from this pressure.

Sam and Jeannine met early in their sophomore year. They formed a strong (and, very quickly, a sexual) attachment to each other. In many ways their relationship was a refuge from their families, but it was also a duplication of their families' intensity. Jeannine got pregnant, and they married. Jeannine's family expressed their upset and displeasure at the marriage by cutting off emotionally, and Jeannine in effect adopted Sam's family as her own.

When the children came, however, Jeannine followed the example of both families by shifting her emotional attachment to the children. She got more distant from her in-laws and from Sam. Meanwhile, Sam's career progressed, with success following upon success. He was first in his class in medical school, became a resident at one of New York's top teaching hospitals, and eventually received an academic appointment there.

As time went on, Jeannine's attachment to and involvement with her children intensified. She wouldn't leave them with anyone to go away with Sam; she spent most of her day volunteering at their school; she talked of little else but them. Sam's sense of self-importance grew, and he became more resentful of Jeannine's sexual distance. He had met Sarah during his residency and two years later began the affair. The triangle became entrenched and had been going on for 10 years when Sam and Jeannine began therapy.

Sam described himself as having been quite competent as a kid. He grew up in Brooklyn, New York, in a mixed cultural environment, with peers who would one day be successful and others who would not. The criteria by which these kids judged themselves and others were academic achievement, which Sam was very good at; athletic competence, where he was only so-so; and sexual successes, of which he had none. Sam didn't totally understand his lack of sexual prowess, but he did know that he was insecure. He feared that he'd be unable to perform—that he would make a fool of himself. He remembers when he struck up a relationship with an intelligent but sexually "easy" young woman whom "everyone" had slept with. He didn't have a sexual relationship with her, but an intellectual one.

Jeannine was a compliant daughter whose first rebellion was her refusal to have the abortion that her attorney father demanded. Her second rebellion was her decision to marry this poor kid with lots of potential.

As the marriage developed, there were many problems and conflicts. They included Jeannine's feelings of being trapped by the pregnancy and her resentment about having to drop out of college. However, there had always been a strong bond between Sam and her. It was exemplified by the fact that Sam could remember exactly what Jeannine had looked like and was wearing the day he met her. Far from saying that it proved Sam saw her as just a sex object, Jeannine thought that it illustrated how caring and attentive he had always been.

Jeannine was exceptional in her ability to acknowledge that Sam's affair had given her relief from his badgering her for sex. In tracking the historical facts, she was able to link the beginnings of Sam and Sarah's relationship with her feelings of relief from Sam's sexual pressure. To this day, Sam remains insecure about his sexual attractiveness in spite of his success in his profession and in spite of feedback about his attractiveness from many women over the years.

As the therapy progressed, Sam confronted his denial of his attachment to and dependence on Jeannine. He realized that he had never really felt his attachment and dependence until the turmoil after the discovery of his affair. When the fear of losing Jeannine surfaced with intensity, he became open to the idea that his extramarital sexual activities were his way of leaving the relationship without having to leave. He came to see it as a way of denying his dependence and behaving in a pseudo independent way. In that sense, this case illustrates the affair triangle as an outgrowth of the emotional fusion in the marriage.[1]

The kind of emotional process within and between individuals

---

[1] See Guerin et al. (1987, pp. 44–50).

that we see in Sam and Jeannine's distance and mutual resentment fuels the activation of triangles, and the repetitive, reactive movement within them. In turn, triangles fuel more reactive emotional process, as Sam's affair with Sarah increased the distance between him and Jeannine. This in turn fortified Jeannine's emotional investment in her children and Sam's in his work. These two interlocking triangles had been set in place for a decade. Thus are structure and process connected.

EMOTIONAL PROCESS AND TRIANGLES

Emotional arousal of almost any kind (anxiety, depression, or intense relationship conflict, for example) can trigger one member of a dyad to turn to a third person for solace, leaving the other member of the dyad in an outsider position. Alternatively, emotional arousal can trigger a third person to move in toward one or both members of a dyad. Once this happens and a triangle is formed, the very existence and activity of the triangle either perpetuate the emotional process that led to the activation of the triangle or trigger new kinds of emotional arousal (e.g., anger, jealousy, suspicion). Because the triangle is dysfunctional and doesn't work, it perpetuates and eventually adds to the emotional intensity. It becomes self-perpetuating, often needing even more triangles to handle the increased intensity. The multiproblem, disorganized family is an example, often ending up surrounded by many agencies: welfare, court, therapy, probation.

There are many theories about the nature of emotional process in triangles. Freud thought that biologically rooted sexual and aggressive impulses accounted for the activation of the oedipal triangle. Bowen taught that the emotional process underlying triangles is fusion. Fogarty focuses on structure and movement, but he has written that the underlying emotional processes are in the individual: anxiety, depression, emptiness, and inner death. Guerin's approach has emphasized the interconnections between structure and process and looks at process in relationships: what goes on (e.g., the transmission of anxiety) in the conduit that connects one person with another. For now we prefer to leave the theoretical question open and continue to listen to what people say about their emotional reactions in triangles.

Let's begin with Bowen's conviction, reinforced by our own and others' clinical and naturalistic observations, that the emotional pro-cess in any dyad is unstable. People usually think of relationships as static: "I don't like my brother and I never have. I avoid him as much as possible." In fact, all relationships have changed over time and will continue to change in the future: "Well, yeah, my brother and I were best friends as kids, but we broke off when I married my wife, even though he warned me not to. We kind of came back together again when our father died, but my wife has never really forgiven him, and so it kind of petered out." Therapists also tend to see relationships as stable. When they see a couple who have been constantly fighting improve after a few therapy sessions, they sometimes assume that a new, friendly stability has replaced the old stability of fighting. They (and the couple) underestimate the cyclical nature of long-term relationships and are not prepared for a return of the bitterness after still more sessions.

Like Bowen[2] and Fogarty,[3] we believe that dyadic instability is tied to people's conflicting needs for autonomy and connection. Efforts to meet these two needs simultaneously result in alternating cycles of separation anxiety and incorporation anxiety.[4] One or both members of the dyad then begin to experience internal discomfort and emotional arousal, and the tension escalates in the relationship. At this point the dyad is set up for the activation of one or more triangles to stabilize the relationship process.

In theory, every individual seeks emotional survival with a minimum of internal discomfort and anxiety. On one hand, most people behave as though survival requires connection with another human being. On the other hand, being tied to another person poses the risk of losing yourself, of being incorporated into the other, of being swallowed up. In other words, the flip side of being connected is being controlled.

Individuals differ in what makes up just the right balance for them between connection and independence, closeness and distance, controlling and being controlled. Everyone spends a good deal of time and energy in his or her relationships trying to find that balance. This means that every dyad is constantly in motion. Both members of the dyad move toward and away from each other, driven by alternating cycles of variably intense separation anxiety and incorporation

---

[2] Bowen (1966; reprinted in Bowen, 1978).

[3] Fogarty (1975).

[4] Bowen (1957; reprinted in Bowen, 1978).

anxiety. This constant, anxious movement is the external marker of relationship fusion and the setup for relationship instability.

What's comfortable for one person depends on which kind of anxiety, separation, or incorporation, predominates for him or her at any particular moment. For an emotional distancer, incorporation anxiety predominates most of the time, and for an emotional pursuer, the most common experience is separation anxiety. Since emotional pursuers and distancers attract one another, it is likely that each person in the twosome will be experiencing the opposite kind of anxiety at any given moment. This is not always true, of course, because the potential for separation anxiety is in every distancer, and the potential for incorporation anxiety is in every pursuer; these feelings will surface in certain contexts or under certain conditions. Nevertheless, because often in any dyad each person feels opposite kinds of anxiety, tension and instability in the twosome are inevitable.

As this tension and instability grow, the two people try to manage their problem either by increased distance or by allowing one to control the other. Exquisite sensitivities develop, and certain issues in the relationship become closed off to discussion. A person experiences wants as needs that the other doesn't meet, and the tension becomes unbearable for both partners, though perhaps to different degrees. At this point, either the distance between the twosome increases, or one adapts to the demands of the other and submits to being controlled. Either way, people's discomfort increases, one person moves toward a third person, and a potential triangle is activated. The alternatives to the activation of a triangle are for both people to work on the issues in the dyad or for the dyad to break up.

The tendency to introduce a third person into the picture is automatic (i.e., reactive, unthinking, emotional)—a response to the instability in a twosome when there is tension, discomfort, frustration, or conflict, and the two people cannot see the underlying difficulty. They concretize it as a problem of sex, children, in-laws, or something else where the core problem does not lie, and therefore they conclude that the solution doesn't lie there either. Or they "know" the solution but it is too painful to face. Thus, a wife may accuse her husband of having an affair, a child may tell his mother that his teacher doesn't like him, a man may tell his sister that their mother is hurt because she sees so little of her mother. These are examples of triangulation by introducing a third party into the conversation between two people. Activating a triangle also occurs when one person in a tense twosome moves to establish a closeness with a third person. This leaves the other person on the outside. One example is a wife who has an affair in response to her husband's lack of sexual interest in her, and he begins to feel nervous and neglected. Another example is an alcoholic husband who attends AA meetings twice a day long after he establishes his sobriety. His wife says things like, "I saw more of him when he was drinking, and I didn't have to listen to all that AA talk." A third example is a child who goes to the second parent whenever the first parent refuses a request.

It is important to remember that activating a triangle is an automatic emotional process and does not imply conscious awareness. Two principles are necessary to remember in this connection. First, the greater the attachment in a twosome, the greater is the potential for reactivity, and so the greater is the potential for the activation of a triangle. Second, a potential triangle, having been established, remains in existence permanently and can be activated and reactivated anytime, or can be duplicated in another generation.

The primary parental triangle (the triangle with one's parents), established when one is a child, is a prime example of these two principles. We are caught in it repeatedly throughout our lives, as it is activated and reactivated under life's stresses. Experience conditions us to repeat its patterns with other people in our lives, notably our spouses and children. Edmund L. was a 38-year-old man whose parents were in their early 60s. As an only child, he had been the apple of his parents' eyes, but he always felt closer to his mother than to his father. His mother was "easier to talk to" and had always been more approving of everything Edmund did than his father. As a child, Edmund remembered, he was "kind of afraid" of his father and tended to avoid him whenever possible. When Edmund was an adolescent and had minor behavioral problems in school, his father was extremely critical and blamed his mother for being too easy on him. After Edmund's graduation from college, his parents divorced, and Edmund gravitated unmistakably to his mother's side. He encouraged her, spent time with her, and listened patiently to her version of the marital problem. He avoided his father, refused to listen to any criticism of his mother, and wouldn't talk with his father's lawyer. During this time Edmund developed ulcerative colitis.

Edmund married at 26, and years later he and his wife, Allison, had a baby boy whom they named Stephen, after Edmund's maternal grandfather. Edmund rarely saw or talked to his father, who had moved from New York to Florida soon after the divorce. However, he sought treatment after a particularly tearful fight with Allison about the time he spent at a boatyard with his buddies. He was concerned that he was "becoming just like my old man." He found, for example, that he was critical of Stephen and getting increasingly distant from him and that he resented Allison's powerful attachment to the boy. The pattern set up in Edmund's primary parental triangle was still dogging him—not just in his relationships with his parents, but in his role as husband and father as well.

Activation (or reactivation) of triangles increases in high-stress situations to produce many interlocking triangles, both inside and outside the family system. Consider what happens when one member of a twosome moves to establish a closeness with a third party and leaves the other on the outside. That person may become so uncomfortable that he or she does the same thing: moves to establish closeness with a fourth person. This activates a second, interlocking, triangle, which can lead to the activation of a third, and so on. For example, suppose a woman feels neglected and uncared for by her husband. She puts her emotional energies into caring for her daughter and gives up on him. He first feels relieved at the reduction in her demands on him and then becomes resentful and blaming. He has an affair. When his wife finds out about it, she calls his mother to complain about him. When the activation of triangles can't contain the discomfort and tension within the family system, outside systems (school, the police, the medical community, therapists) are triangled in.

What is a therapist to do in the face of this constant triangling by individuals, couples, and families? Murray Bowen said that the only way to break the cycle of triangulation is for the therapist, or a well-coached family member, to stay in emotional contact with both members of the original twosome while holding his or her own reactivity in check and not to take sides with either of the other two. If someone does this, the emotional reactivity within the twosome will automatically decrease. The stage will be set for them to deal with the issues in that relationship without triangling.

One key to staying out of triangles is not to side with one person against the other. Some therapists do this by not taking any positions, or by refusing to answer specific questions, or by not making their positions clear when asked about specific issues in the family. Unfortunately, this fear of being in a triangle can serve to paralyze therapists, who often fail to discriminate between neutrality and no-self waffling. In clinical work, "neutrality" means *emotional* neutrality or nonreactivity to a patient's or family member's behavior, feelings, or beliefs. It *doesn't* mean refusing to say anything, or saying the equivalent of "You're not going to get me in a triangle."

Ideally, when therapists decide to take positions on matters of therapeutic relevance, those positions have everything to do with fact-based observations about what works in families and relationships and what doesn't, and little to do with the therapist's emotionally charged beliefs on issues of the day, or philosophical, theological, and other perspectives on life. This allows for respectful differences of opinion and levels of psychotherapeutic influence that are appropriate to the mutual undertaking of therapy. For example, the opinions of the therapist on abortion, divorce, and sexual ethics are less relevant to the therapeutic process than the therapist's fact-based observations about the importance of respect and taking responsibility for one's own feelings and behavior.

Still, there are issues that, for the therapist to be in control of the therapeutic process, the therapist must be clear about. They include violence, intimidation, and violations of sexual boundaries. Therapy cannot go on in a positive direction while threats of physical and emotional abuse or violation of sexual boundaries are continuing to happen. It is imperative for the therapist to be able to take firm positions about the unacceptability of this type of behavior and the importance of controlling it before attempting to understand the underlying dynamics. In this way the therapist can take an appropriate stance, maintain control of the process, and operate with a clear boundary between what is the therapist's personal material and that which is therapeutically relevant.

Working on yourself and your own family gives you a healthy respect for the omnipresence, the subtlety, and the problems of triangulation. Then you can take positions based on principles that you believe in without being caught in a therapy triangle. Of course, your presentation of these principles will vary from case to case and from time to time, depending on such factors as the emotional climate at the moment and the solidity of the therapeutic relationship with a particular patient or family member at a given time. Nevertheless, belief in the principle (e.g., that each member of a family is responsible for his or her own feelings) remains constant.

As a therapist, you need to learn to recognize signs that you are vulnerable to being caught in a triangle. These signs will vary from one therapist to another, but generic signs include running out of questions to ask (your model fosters the use of continuous process questions, but the tension in the room is so high that you're losing your grip on your model), a feeling that the clock is moving very slowly (you may be anxious and less able to stay clear of the family process—or it could just be that this is the 10th family today), irritation within the therapist, a desire not to see this patient, anger with the patient and a desire to change him or her, and not to listen or pursue understanding. Signs more specific to particular therapists happen when the issues being dealt with (e.g., divorce, sexual abuse, parental neglect of children) are by a matter of historical fact issues in the therapist's own family system.

This *in situ* therapeutic detriangling is a necessary precondition for further experimental moves. It lowers emotional arousal in the individuals and creates a clarity of thinking that allows them to be accessible to coaching about the way they form triangles and act in them. With emotional arousal reduced, the therapist can teach people not to make the moves they have always made in forming triangles but, instead, to try different moves. We can combine such structural experiments with reflection on the emotional process that has been part of the triangles over time or on the process that gets uncovered because of these new moves (process experiments).

An example of a structural experiment in a triangle with children would be the old family therapy prescription of moving the mother out and father in. Recall Sam—the surgeon who couldn't decide whether to leave his wife for his lover—and Jeannine, for instance. If the therapist decided to work on the interlocking triangle with their children, Sam might be encouraged to spend more time with his children and take more responsibility for their upbringing. Simultaneously, Jeannine would be encouraged to pull back from the children and focus on another aspect of her life. This alteration of the structure of the triangle would surface dyadic and individual process that would then be discussed and dealt with.

Feminists have criticized this strategy because the way therapists implement it often implies that the mother–child enmeshment is the mother's fault and that moving the father in is "privileging patriarchy."[5] It's best to stay aware of the potential for sending a sexist message here. You can sometimes clarify your intentions by scheduling a separate appointment with the mother to explain your thinking more clearly and answer questions about what you're up to. You emphasize that you imply no blame and that when you're dealing with difficult

---

[5] Luepnitz (1988).

emotional problems you're just looking for something that will work. You can point out that you're pulling the mother back because her husband won't move into his fathering position until she is out of sight. Trying it the other way around mostly *doesn't work.* Anyway, it's a temporary move and will give the father a living experience of how difficult being the more involved parent is. You're saying that the mother's biggest asset is herself, and by pulling back, she is using herself rather than trying to change her husband in his fathering.

A process experiment might be indicated in its own right when a structural experiment is contraindicated or impossible or when a structural experiment surfaces a process that we must deal with. In Sam and Jeannine's case, a process experiment might go something like this: Sam complains of Jeannine's sexual distance, and Jeannine replies that Sam is too critical for her to be interested in making love with him. The therapist might think that Sam's criticism is an indirect expression of his anger about sex, that the criticism further distances Jeannine, and that the circle goes on like that. The therapist might suggest a process experiment in which Sam refrains from critical comments about his wife, which, Sam may discover, increases his inner turmoil. The inner turmoil gets communicated across the relationship, which has the same effect as the criticism: Jeannine distances. The next phase of the experiment would be for Sam to modulate and manage his inner tension so that he doesn't transmit it. By cognitive effort, or by medication, or by sublimation, or by another mechanism, Sam succeeds in managing his upset. In response, Jeannine does not move toward Sam, but insists he is still critical and upset with her. If Jeannine cannot document this and Sam really has managed his anxiety better, the experiment now shows that Sam's upset and criticism have served some function for Jeannine. Perhaps it has helped her avoid intimacy, avoid her anger, or avoid dealing with her long-term upset about the cutoff from her family.

This chapter and the previous one have dealt with the structure of triangles, the emotional processes that occur in them, and the functions they serve for individuals, dyads, and relationship systems. In the next chapter we show how structure, process, and function work together.

CHAPTER SIX

The Interaction of Structure, Process, and Function

THE RELATIONSHIP OF STRUCTURE AND PROCESS

The activation of a triangle is like flipping a circuit breaker to "on" in an electrical system: Now there is a conduit for emotional energy to move back and forth among the people in the triangle. The energy moves in a way that obstructs any genuine one-on-one relationship for the participants in the triangle. This energy is the fuel for dysfunctional movement in the triangle. The triangle's underlying emotional process drives the dysfunctional movement—a process that is usually out of awareness. The underlying process comes into awareness in therapy as people try different (detriangling) moves in the reconstruction of triangles.

To understand the emotional circuitry in a triangle, it's necessary to remember that each of the three persons involved will either be seeking closeness with one of the other two or trying to avoid tension by seeking distance in periods of stress. The emotional energy in the triangle fuels people's movements toward or away from one another (thus affecting the triangle's structure), and these moves in turn produce emotional reactions that are the fuel for further moves, and so on.

When people present for treatment, this interplay between emotional process and structure has become fixed. It locks the people involved into the same repetitive moves, countermoves, and emotional reactions. This is the first element of triangulation. When people make different moves, perhaps as an experiment suggested in therapy, new emotional reactions take place. These represent the underlying emotional process that needs to be dealt with in the dyads and individuals that make up the triangle. This underlying emotional process is the second element of triangulation.

The emotional process of triangles is about attachment, influence, or both. It was Sam's upset over Jeannine's attachment to the children, and his disappointed expectation that she would be primarily attached to him, that sparked his movement toward an affair with Sarah (pp. 82–85). Learning that the primacy of Sam's sexual attachment had shifted away from her to Sarah prompted Jeannine's move toward therapy. Expectations are always present in any twosome about where the primacy of attachment and influence will lie. In three interconnected twosomes (a potential triangle), these expectations can easily conflict. For example, a husband expects that his wife will listen to him when it comes to deciding the inheritance she received from her paternal grandmother. The wife's father believes that she should listen to him. After all, the money came from his mother, and he has always guided his daughter when it comes to money. If this potential triangle was not already active, it will become active when they read the will.

Think again about the rubber band wound around the three people. A change in the position of one will necessarily create a change in the position of the others, or an increased tension between them. The rubber band will keep the sum of the distances among the three people at a constant figure. If one moves away, the other two will pull closer to each other. It is this rubber-band effect that keeps the system from breaking, but it is also very limiting.

Overloaded emotionality in each of the three twosomes is partly transferred into another twosome. The result is a dilution and confusion of the emotional issues and tensions. There is still an overload of tension in the system, but it shifts around. It may appear as conflict in any one twosome or as symptoms in any member.

At this point, the triangle takes on a life of its own. It becomes larger than the sum of its parts. Triangulation is a process that rises above and dominates the three people and their relationships. As the rubber band takes over, movement in one necessarily accompanies movement in the other person or relationship. Self-determination, the ability of any one person to decide and direct his or her own movement, gives way to reactive movement. The freedom of each person is limited. Thus, the triangle runs the three people even if they aren't aware of it.

If therapy is directed at restructuring the triangle by getting one or more individuals to make different moves within it, a different emotional process will emerge. Imagine, for example, that a mother has been giving most of her attention and nurturance to her daughter and distancing from her husband and that the husband has been a workaholic for years. The resulting emotional process has had the mother angry with her husband and admiring of her daughter, and the father has become intensely critical of mother and child. The therapist coaches the mother to pull back from her daughter and to focus on her relationship with a sister from whom she cut herself off. He coaches the father to move toward his daughter and assume more responsibility for her care. As they carry out these moves, both parents experience new emotional reactions: The mother becomes depressed, and the father feels inadequate. The feelings of depression and inadequacy in these two individuals are, we assume, the underlying process that must be addressed. The mother's focus on the child allowed her to avoid her depression, and the father's focus on work kept his lifelong feelings of inadequacy at bay. It is the work on the triangles that has surfaced that process and made it accessible.

MECHANISMS OF TRIANGLE ACTIVATION

Three people who have a history of having been in an active triangle are vulnerable to being a triangle again if stress becomes sufficiently high. Stress triggers the activation of potential triangles. Individuals move toward and away from one another driven by their need to calm anxiety or emotional arousal. Given the emotional process that sets up the potential for triangles, the activation of a triangle requires the cooperation of all three people (or groups of people) involved. All of them have three movement options: to move away, to move in, or to stand still. We can describe the way triangles are activated by looking from the viewpoint of any one of the three people and of how they move.

1. *One person in a tense dyad moves toward a third person, leaving the other person in the original dyad in the outside position.* An affair is an obvious example of this mechanism. One spouse moves toward an outsider in an emotionally intense way so that the other spouse is left out, feeling alone and uncared for. Another example is a son who talks to his older sister about his anger at his younger brother, increasing the

distance and lack of connection between his brother and him. The same sort of thing happens a lot in the workplace, when an unhappy worker moans to a coworker about their supervisor instead of talking directly with the supervisor about the issues. During the early days of consciousness raising in the 1960s, women would sometimes get together and bond around their frustration and anger with the men in their lives. The commiseration helped women feel less alone, but often their upset never got dealt with in their relationships with those men.

2. *One person in a tense dyad isolates him- or herself enough to push the other member of the dyad and a third person together.* An example of this would be the workaholic husband whose wife begins devoting most of her time and emotional energy to her child (or her parent, or her sister). Another example would be a seriously ill family member who is very involved in treatment and health issues. The patient's family members don't want to upset the patient, so they avoid the subject with the patient and talk among themselves about their concern for him or her. Still another version of this category might be an angry, distant adolescent avoiding the family while his parents walk on eggshells and worry with one another but don't take the adolescent on.

3. *A third person moves in toward one or both members of a tense dyad.* An example of this mechanism is the mother who, after finding out from her daughter that the daughter's marriage is in trouble, tries to act as mediator and advisor to one or both of the spouses. (This is invariably a triangle. People can't act as mediators in their own families without being caught. A parent trying to mediate a child's marriage is different from a therapist in the same situation because the therapist has no emotional investment in the outcome. If the therapist were to have an emotional investment, that would set up a therapy triangle.) Another example that we all recognize is the parent who can't let his or her children settle their disagreements and needs to intervene like King Solomon. This category is also very popular with therapists in their own families. Most of us have a hard time leaving the people we love to resolve their own disputes and problems.

These are the three basic mechanisms of triangle activation, and they vary according to the positive or negative polarity of the movement that occurs in them. For example, Joyce and Dan K. called for an appointment shortly after Joyce discovered that Dan had been involved in an affair for the past 6 months. (He had left two ticket stubs for a rock concert in his jacket pocket. Joyce found them and confronted Dan with his story that he had been at the office that evening.) Dan was a 41-year-old middle manager who was changing jobs. He had been a diabetic since age 15, but he wasn't responsible about caring for himself. His mother, and then his wife, had taken much of the responsibility for watching out for Dan's health. He would do things like go out running without carrying emergency glucose tablets and then collapse. Joyce would find him sprawled on the side of the road and get an ambulance to take him to the hospital. Dan's mother, whom he idealized, had died 2 years earlier, and his expectations that Joyce would take care of him now increasingly irritated her. His mother's death and the prospect of changing jobs had Dan in a state of high anxiety. Joyce, while a caretaker, had always been sexually and emotionally distant. Dan described her as unresponsive in bed, reluctant to initiate or accept physical displays of affection, and stingy with praise. His involvement with the woman with whom he was having the affair made him feel "wonderful."

Sometimes therapy itself can illustrate a variation in the way triangles are activated: Both people in a reactive dyad move toward a third person (the therapist) to stabilize their relationship. George and Loretta J. were a couple in their 50s who had been married for 20 years. Their marriage fluctuated between periods of moderate closeness and angry distance. They reported that the amplitude of these fluctuations had been growing in recent years. They were increasingly frightened that some day the distance and anger would get so bad that one of them would give up and get a divorce. They came to therapy in the hope that the therapist would save their marriage, but they stated in the first meeting that neither was interested in digging too deeply into any individual problems. As therapy progressed, the couple found ways of avoiding several painful but important issues. Eventually, it became clear that George expected the therapist to talk to Loretta and get her to stop the behavior he didn't like. Loretta expected the same: The therapist would talk to George and get him to change.

We could call another variant the "peacemaker" mechanism. In cases like this, the conflict in a dyad incorporates, or "hooks," a third person, who moves in to stabilize the dyad. Al G. and Jill H. are a young engaged couple who report that they have many problems with each other. Al complains most bitterly about Jill's mother, who is constantly interfering. She is apparently hypervigilant about any conflict between Al and her daughter and moves in immediately to give advice. According to Al, most of the advice is directed at how Al could improve his treatment of Jill. Jill insists that her mother is equally tough on her. Both report that, the more they avoid her, the more Jill's mother is showing signs of depression.

Another variation, the acting-out mechanism, is illustrated by a child who is sensitive to the upset of one parent and doesn't even realize it. As this child senses that parent's anxiety, she or he begins to act out and becomes the focus of both parents' concern. Abbie F. was a 15-year-old young woman who had been admitted to the psychiatric ward of a community hospital for evaluation following a suicide attempt by swallowing a half-bottle of her mother's Xanax. This suicide attempt was the latest in what her parents said was an escalating pattern of troubled behavior. Abbie's mother was seen alone and asked why she takes Xanax. She reported that she had been feeling depressed and had had difficulty falling asleep in the year since her father died. Asked about any more recent stressors, she admitted that she hadn't been feeling sexual during that time either and that she is afraid her husband might be having an affair.

FIGURING OUT FUNCTION

It is the dialectic between the attractiveness of stability and the need for change that we are dealing with when we speak of the function of triangles. Triangles provide stability to relationship systems, but they impede the working out of conflicts.

Once you start noticing triangles, either clinically or in your everyday relationships, you'll begin to notice that triangles serve at least three functions for any relationship system: containment of tension, displacement of conflict, and avoidance of intimacy in the dyadic relationship.

The containment of tension can be illustrated by Tom E., a 50-year-old lawyer, Andrea, his social worker wife, and their daughter, Deirdre, a sophomore at a college 2 hours from home. Deirdre was their only child, and both Tom and Andrea were extremely attached to her. When she was away at school, Tom and Andrea were mildly depressed, socialized very little with friends, and their conversations were almost always about Deirdre. Their tension was close to the surface and was managed by distance and involvement in work. When Deirdre was home, by contrast, Tom and Andrea were noticeably brighter in mood. The three of them went on vacation and did things together such as going to dinner and to the movies. Deirdre sensed their need for her and was ambivalent about it. She wanted to become independent, but she was afraid of it for herself and worried about her parents. Conversations revolved around a variety of topics—politics, literature, and the activities of Deirdre and her many friends. The triangle with Deirdre provided stability to Tom and Andrea's relationship, but it put off the necessity of dealing with the tensions between them and with the many issues of each one's middle-aged life. Maybe we ought to call the "empty-nest syndrome" the "two-legged stool syndrome."

Jack C. and Keith D. illustrate the displacement of conflict function. They were colleagues and friends who worked as department managers in a large corporation in metropolitan New York. They shared such interests as sports cars and college basketball; the company had hired them at approximately the same time, and they had risen through the corporate ranks in remarkably symmetrical fashion. They joked and jousted with one another about many things—except their competitiveness with each other. This topic somehow was off limits, although their to-the-death tennis matches were the talk of the company picnic every year. Keith might be found sneaking a peek at the performance statistics of Jack's department 10 days before they were published. Jack might be observed timing the length of a meeting between Keith and the divisional vice-president.

The clerical staff knew enough not to challenge their denial about their competitiveness, and they joined in the conspiracy to keep it underground. However, underground process usually finds its way to the surface. In this case, it materialized only through their dealings with an administrative assistant who had worked at various times for both of them. Jack had sometimes asked her to work late, and she usually refused. Once he had pressed her to complete a task more quickly than usual, and she failed to meet his deadline. Keith had never asked this assistant for extra work and had invariably been satisfied with the work she did do. Jack's frustration with her had been expressed by urging Keith to agree to fire her; Keith would reply that Jack was expecting too much and overreacting. Thus they had displaced the conflict between them onto the issue of the assistant, and they never dealt with the real issue between them, their competition with each other.

An obvious example of the avoidance of intimacy function is the extramarital affair. In many of these cases, the spouse who has an affair is in denial about his or her powerful dependence on and attachment to the other spouse. Having an affair is often a way to "leave without leaving": to deny the dependence and attachment, and act as if they didn't exist, but without dealing functionally with the reality of these emotions. The same process often occurs, apparently more innocently, when one partner starts spending all of his or her free time with a friend. They share confidences, talk about things they talk about with no one else, and don't tell their spouses. It's as if they have a secret life.

If you want to understand the functions of triangles, you have to make some conceptual distinctions.

1. *Function as a positive consequence.* "The function of the heart is to pump oxygenated and nutrient-laden blood to the rest of the body." This kind of statement says, in effect, that the beneficial, indeed essential, consequence of the heart's action is that the body is supplied with necessary nutrition. "The functions of this extramarital affair are to relieve the sexual pressure on the wife of the husband's demands and to meet the husband's sexual needs." This kind of statement says that an extramarital affair can have positive consequences for individuals or a dyad.

2. *Positive for whom?* "The function of managed care is to lower health care costs." This statement, while accurate when applied to insurance companies and premium payers, ignores the *negative* consequences for medical professionals and hospitals, whose incomes and autonomy decrease, and for the patients who are discharged "quicker and sicker." "The function of the triangle between a recovering alcoholic, his sponsor, and his wife is that the connection between husband and sponsor allows the husband to stay sober." This statement, while accurate, does not address the negative consequences of the triangle on the wife, who is now in the outsider position, or on the marriage, which may be undermined because of it.

3. *Negative consequences.* These are best understood as dysfunctions. "The function of a parent–child triangle is that it allows the spouses/parents to avoid the real issues between them." This statement, at least from some perspectives, is a statement of the negative consequence of a triangle. Avoiding the real issues is probably a bad idea for everyone involved. Thus, perhaps a better phrasing would be, "The *dys*function of this triangle. .ÿ20.ÿ20."

For individuals, the function served by triangles is that triangles enable people to calm their anxiety by achieving closeness or avoiding relationship tension. Although these effects are only temporary, the need for closeness or the discomfort of tension is so great that people move automatically to triangles.

For twosomes, triangles serve to dilute or confuse the issues between the two people and allow them to avoid those issues. By lowering tension, triangles prevent the twosome from breaking up. These effects, too, are temporary, but continually creating new triangles can prolong them.

For larger systems, such as whole families, triangles encapsulate and project system problems or issues and so serve a homeostatic function. Triangles enable systems to survive without change. We assume that this function, too, works only temporarily, although it may last for a very long time—even across many generations—until collapse is imminent.

From a clinical point of view, observing the functions that triangles serve raises the issue of whether we should always eliminate triangles when we discover them in therapy. Perhaps a particular triangle is a necessary element in the solution of a problem. It may be, as it were, a crutch that people need as they work toward a long-term solution to their problems.

The word "function" can be used in many different ways. It usually suggests a purpose, such as performing its normal action. For example, the purpose of the automobile engine is to propel the car along the highway. The purpose of the heart is to propel blood through the circulatory system. These are the proper actions for which these objects are fitted.

Function can also mean, "Does it function? Does it work, and how well does it work?" Here people employ the term to define how well something meets its purpose. "Is the heart pumping well, and can the motor move the car along the highway?" It is a functional or dysfunctional family system, heart, or motor. Does it operate or perform successfully or effectively?

These definitions raise thorny questions. What is a normal action or a proper purpose? What is the unit that we should study to see if the object or person is performing successfully? When it comes to objects, the answers to these questions are simple and clear. When it comes to people, the answers are not so simple or clear.

If we call something normal, what does that mean, and who sets the norm? For many years, the American Psychiatric Association called homosexuality abnormal and then by a vote decided that it was no longer abnormal. Does normal mean conforming to the way most people are, or to the popular culture, and does it change accordingly? Does it mean the usual, or that which is natural? If blowing one's top when one is hurt is natural, is this the normal reaction, and furthermore, is it functional, or is the "normal" reaction here a *dys*functional reaction? Is doing what comes naturally functional or even normal? If you hurt me and I strike back and seriously injure you, I may have reacted naturally and normally, but do we want to encourage this kind of natural, normal behavior? If we consider the word "proper," we add more complications. Does proper mean the ordinary, or the moral, or the expected response or activity, or does it simply mean the pragmatic "it works" response or action? Again, who decides these standards?

- Mrs. A. is a 40-year-old woman with panic disorder manifested by many symptoms of anxiety such as chest pain and fear of fainting. These symptoms occurred most often when she was driving on the highway. Otherwise, the panic disorder was not particularly bothersome to her as a homemaker. She decided to adjust to it, to limit her driving to local destinations, and did not experience any more panic attacks.
- Mrs. A. is a 40-year-old homemaker with panic attacks. She went into therapy, was placed on medication, and experienced no more panic attacks. She often wonders if she cured the disorder, or if the medication did, and sometimes she gets concerned that the panic will return.
- Mrs. A. goes to a marriage counselor who identifies the panic as fear of abandonment by her mother when she was growing up and now by her husband. She is afraid of being left alone. After much work, her husband cuts down on his tennis and golf, and Mrs. A. feels better, with much less anxiety. Nevertheless, now her husband feels depressed as if he had lost something.
- Mrs. and Mr. A. and their two children enter family therapy. Mrs. A. now feels much better since everybody is sharing the responsibility of family life, and the therapist agrees that all should do this. Mr. A., however, feels constrained, and the children feel angry, as if the parents should solve their own problems. The last thing in the world the children need is another parent (the therapist).
- Mrs. A. joins a religious group founded on AA principles and

decides to turn those things in her life that she cannot control over to God. She feels fine, but her husband is upset over her frequent absences from home to attend evening and weekend meetings.

Apparently, with good intentions, people will differ in their standards and will differ at different times in their lives. Standards of judgment are therefore much more emotional than most of us would like to believe. If every judgment is a judgment of people, motivation, situations, and complex interactions over a continuum, things are clearest at both ends of the continuum. As one moves toward the center, vision becomes blurred and judgment grayer. The continuum is black and white at the extremes and grayer toward the center where most events occur. Other complications include, "Who sets the standards?" Another major factor in the mental health field is the unit of study. Does one assess improved function by surveying the individual, or the personal relationship (the twosome), or the family system?

If a wife loses her panic symptoms and her husband is now acting out his angry responses, is that an improvement? The answer depends on the field of vision one is using. If a husband is having an affair and is trying to stabilize a marriage by doing so, is that an improvement over divorce? If a man is drinking to keep from looking at certain feelings, is that a dysfunction? Or would he kill himself to avoid those feelings if he didn't drink? If the alcohol makes him feel better and his wife is worse, is that functional or dysfunctional; is it better or worse? If a man is having an affair to keep the marriage together, then the triangle is serving its purpose if the wife doesn't find out about the affair. But is the affair functional? Would it be more functional if he worked on the marriage so that the affair was unnecessary? It turns out that the terms function and functional are formidably complicated. Let's try to sort some out some of the complexity.

Triangles and Dysfunction

Triangles usually overload problems onto one person and excuse others. They are built on reactivity that puts blinders on the observation of self. They therefore decrease the freedom of self to move with options and freely in a system. Because they displace issues, they obscure underlying process in superficial issues and images. None of this is conducive to differentiation or fulfillment.

Function and Functional

The purpose (function) of triangles is to stabilize the twosome. This often works temporarily, but all too often it ends up creating more difficulties. Therefore it doesn't work (is not functional) after a while. The triangle doesn't work because the twosome is both the greatest test of differentiation and the closest that one can come to fulfillment. This is an assumption based on romantic love, intimacy, monogamy. Even with all breakups and divorces, American society remains stubbornly a "couple" society.

What Is Functional?

Since people will clearly differ over a wide spectrum about what is normal and about what is proper, and since what works for one might not work for another, what "works" is a complicated question. From an individual point of view it is clearer. The symptom is gone. From a systems point of view, we are left with this definition of the workable: The family (or the unit of study) says, "This is a pretty good family (group) to belong to over time." At any given moment, complications arise because no significant change occurs without suffering and pain. Change is a necessary part of life. It happens whether we want it or not. Triangles are attempts to preserve homeostasis in the face of the reality of change. The tension between the search for homeostasis inside self and in personal relationships, and this inevitable change in the system, creates anxiety, stress, and triangles. The path to functional relationships is littered with suffering.

As you've probably discovered, the more you know and learn, the larger the gray area of life becomes, and the extremes of the continuum at either end become smaller, clearer, and firmer. Since most of us operate largely within the gray areas, different people are bound to evaluate life differently, especially on issues such as the normal or the proper or the functional.

Another issue that makes it complicated to talk of function and the functional is the view or philosophy of life that different people have. To some the purpose of life is to live without depression or anxiety. To others, life is a continuum in which depression and anxiety are inevitable as part of the human condition. To them, life is a continuum in which an unspecified amount of these feelings is necessary and exists to keep us honest. They exist, not as problems to get rid of but as opportunities to learn. Even in this group, opinions will vary about when, if ever, these emotional symptoms become problems or signs of mental illness. As usual, these issues are clearer at the extremes but become more confusing as they move toward the median.

Most people who have bothered to think about it would agree to the existence of something that we might term a relationship triangle. They have watched their mother struggle with an extramarital affair, their two older brothers exclude them from a touch football game, their best friend steal their boyfriend. However, they wouldn't necessarily buy into the need for a theoretical consideration of the impact of these phenomena on their emotional and relationship lives. We believe, based on clinical and personal experience, that an understanding and evolution of a conceptual framework for triangles dramatically improve the ability of an individual to work her or his way through the tangled, triangular underbrush to some semblance of operational emotional freedom. It is in the service of this belief that we have tried to formulate and present a theoretical model. Let's turn now to more specifically clinical considerations.

This chapter has defined a working model for that amorphous, molecular movement that goes on in the relationship space between two individuals and then within the structure of a relationship triangle. In addition, this chapter has addressed, as an outgrowth of relationship process, the *function* that a triangle or set of interlocking triangles serves for a relationship system. We have offered some examples of relationship experiments and maneuvers to assist therapists in exposing covert emotional process that is embedded in key relationship triangles. This more clinical focus is the heart of the remaining chapters.

CHAPTER SEVEN

Introducing Triangles in Individual Therapy

For 20 years we've been teaching our students about triangles. The triangle as a relationship structure and triangulation as the reactive emotional process within that structure have been easy ideas for students and therapists to grasp. However, as we sat at many meetings to write about triangles and triangulation for this book, we discovered that these ideas were infinitely more complicated than we had foreseen. There were disagreements about membership in a triangle; whether we could include groups of people such as the members of an extended family in the triangle as a group; whether objects could replace people as one leg of the triangle. Could alcohol be a leg of the triangle? Could issues such as morality serve as the leg of a triangle? Was a triangle always destructive, or did it, in certain circumstances, manage to hold an individual or group together even if in a dysfunctional way? Would things be worse if the triangle didn't exist? Was talking about a third person always an example of triangulation, or could it simply be gossip? Was the signature of a triangle that two people were avoiding looking at each other and at the problems between them?

We came to realize that all these uncertainties and more made it difficult to help students and therapists to see triangles and triangulation in the family in front of them, to avoid being triangled themselves, and to develop mastery of treatment planning. In response to this problem, Guerin began in 1981[1] to develop a clinical typology

---

[1]Described in Guerin and Gordon (1984).

of triangles based on symptom presentation. In 1987,[2] a classification of triangles surrounding marital conflict was added to a previously developed classification of adolescent- and child-focused triangles. In this and the following chapters we refine these two existing typologies of triangles. We also introduce an additional grouping of triangles centered on the problems of coaching and systems psychotherapy of the individual adult.

The development of this triangle typology with its three categories—marital triangles, child and adolescent triangles, and triangles of the individual adult—comes from thousands of clinical hours of working with people from all walks of life who have sought help for varying degrees of individual distress and relationship conflict. Sometimes their presenting problems have explicitly included an active, "hot" triangle. At other times they complain of dyadic conflict or their own internal emotional turmoil. You've probably noticed that there's usually a connection between people's internal storm and relationship conflict. The emotional process that drives this connection automatically drives the formation of relationship triangles.

The triangle typology we propose is constructed on two axes. The first axis is the presenting problem. The presenting problem could be a marital conflict, or a child or adolescent problem. It could also be the problem of an adult individual who comes to therapy alone, either because he or she wants it that way or because his or her spouse won't participate. The second axis is whether the third person in the triangle is outside the multigenerational family system (an "extrafamilial triangle") or a member of the multigenerational family system (an "intrafamilial triangle"). This gives us six types of triangles; for example, marital intrafamilial or adult individual extrafamilial (see Table 7 1). Each of these six types has several commonly seen subtypes, some of which we discuss briefly and exemplify in this chapter and the ones to follow.

This typology is useful to the practicing clinician because it provides a checklist. Such a list alerts her or him to the triangles that are always present but are sometimes concealed in the presentation of symptoms. We hope that the typology will be used to help the therapist think about triangles and watch for them in any clinical situation. *Depending on how the case presents,* the appropriate column in Table 7.1 can be checked to remind therapists of what extrafamilial and

---

[2]Guerin, Fay, Burden, and Kautto (1987).

TABLE 7.1. Triangle Types and Subtypes

	Marital triangles	Child or adolescent triangles	Adult individual triangles

Extra-familial triangles	Extramarital affairs
	Social network
	   triangles
	Occupational
	   triangles
		School-related
		   triangles
		Social network/
		   peer triangles
			Social network
			   triangles
			Occupational
			   triangles

Intra-familial triangles	*Family of origin*
	In-law triangles
	Primary parental
	   triangles
	Nuclear family
	Child-centered
	   triangles
		Family of origin
		Three-generational
		   triangles
		Nuclear family
		Symptomatic
		   child triangles
		Target child
		   triangles
		Parent and sibling
		   triangles
		Sibling subsystem
		   triangles
		Stepfamily triangles
			Family of origin
			Primary parental
			   triangles
			Dysfunctional
			   spouse triangles
			Sibling subsystem
			   triangles
			Nuclear family
			Spouse and
			   child triangles

intrafamilial triangles they most commonly see in that kind of presentation. This gives the therapist some concrete things to look for. Thus, if an adult individual comes in with, for example, depression, the clinician may work for symptom relief by prescribing a course of medication. However, patients get optimal and long-lasting relief from depression only if they also deal with the underlying emotional process. Since this underlying emotional process is itself often triangular in nature, or the route to getting at that process is by focusing on a symptomatic triangle, we must also pay close attention to references the patient makes to other people in her or his life. If the clinician is looking for triangles and hears these sorts of references, she or he will begin to ask questions that will reveal the triangle's structure and bring its emotional process into the open.

As we begin this part of the book, we want to be clear about what we are doing in offering a typology of triangles. Our typology is clinically based. That is, we have chosen to construct a "file" of types of triangles that commonly present in various kinds of clinical situations. We hope this allows the clinician to find more easily the most commonly occurring triangles, to recognize the forms they take and the processes that exist within them, and to have available ways of intervening with them.

The essential points for you to keep in mind as a practicing clinician are: If you're seeing marital conflict, look for these triangles; if you're seeing child-focused family problems, look for these; if you're seeing anxiety, depression, or another dysfunction in an individual, look for these.

USING TRIANGLES IN INDIVIDUAL THERAPY

Individual patients come to you looking for relief from their pain, resolution of their conflicts, and validation that their perceptions are at least somewhat accurate—that they are in fact not crazy. When Richard H. came to therapy, he was experiencing considerable amounts of anxiety. He brought along a 230-page journal filled with episodes from his work life and his marriage that had caused him consternation and emotional pain. He sat down and started to read it, and the therapist listened. The experience was unique, and the content was fascinating, rich in stories that supported the thesis that Richard was star-crossed—born, as it were, to be the exemplar of bad things happening to good people. After 50 minutes of just listening, the therapist ended the session and scheduled another appointment. Since it was the therapist's last appointment for the day, therapist and patient left the office building together. As they walked out, they were caught in a sudden cloudburst, leading the therapist to think his patient might have a point.

At age 39, Richard was a partner in a major accounting firm. During treatment, he and the therapist worked together in defining what was real and what was a manifestation of the patient's abundant obsessional anxiety. In addition, the therapist encouraged Richard to reverse his isolation and repeople his world. Since his marriage and the arrival of his two sons, Richard had been overdosing on work.

As you might predict, Richard was diligent about the work on his cognitive distortions and took the therapist's suggestions seriously—sometimes too seriously. Somehow a too-compliant patient seeking to please can be harder to challenge than a resistant one who specializes in oppositionalism. Several sessions after being nudged to stop isolating himself, Richard reported an upcoming business trip and his plan to take some time to visit his old master sergeant from his time in the Marine Corps. Richard returned 2 weeks later looking well but holding himself in a different way. When he moved, he seemed to be experiencing some bodily discomfort. When the therapist asked about it, Richard wove a fascinating tale of his reunion meeting. He had taken his sergeant out to dinner. While at dinner Richard had inhaled some balsamic vinegar with a bite of salad. He had a laryngospasm, a choking sensation, and a temporary inability to vocalize. His sergeant, alert to the signs and a "can-do" guy, immediately got up, came around the table, and administered the Heimlich maneuver. The laryngospasm passed, but the two broken ribs remained.

Throughout therapy, the therapist tried to balance listening to these fascinating stories and concentrating on the work at hand. Sometimes he could use the stories as material for helping Richard distinguish between what was real and what anxious distortion. Tales of his time with the master sergeant evoked reminiscences of a certain ritual that Richard had exhibited during his time in the Corps. He was able then to reveal in therapy daily rituals that he had denied when asked during the initial evaluation. This disclosure, and the fact that Richard had had only about a 40% improvement in his symptoms, moved the therapist to prescribe Anafranil, a tricyclic antidepressant especially effective with obsessive–compulsive behavior. Over a period of 6 to 8 weeks, the medication raised the level of his symptom relief to about 70%. The therapist was able to document a considerable decrease in the frequency and intensity of Richard's rituals and of his generalized obsessive anxiety. His chronic dysthymic dreams faded, his relationship with his sons improved, and his social life increased. His marriage to Rona was less pressured and negative, but she remained distant, critical, and preoccupied with almost everything but Richard. She was impressed with his improvement, however, and was willing to join the therapy.

At the first joint session Rona validated Richard's progress. "Yes, he's a lot better now, I guess." The therapist challenged her on her sustained distance and seeming indifference to him in spite of the progress and probed for evidence of hurt and resentment accumulated over the years. Rona spoke of the weariness that Richard's obsessiveness and negativity had produced in her, but she denied intense feelings of hurt, anger, or resentment. When the therapist asked whether Rona thought that Richard had been born this way or his mother had made him this way, Rona sighed deeply and wove her own tale. Richard had canonized his mother as a saint in his own mind, but she had never accepted Rona, even after the boys were born. The presence of her brother had blocked Rona's connection with her own mother, and Rona had wished for a closeness with her mother-in-law. Richard interrupted at that point, became defensive, and pleaded the case of his mother who was now 6 years dead.

The medical relief of many symptoms of Richard's anxiety allowed therapy to refocus on the relationships in Richard's life, and this shift led to the emergence of the key triangles. The central triangle involved Richard, Rona, and Richard's sainted mother. The genesis of this triangle went all the way back to the beginning of their marriage when Richard had been unable to make the shift in the primacy of his attachment from his mother to his wife.

Over the next 6 months, Richard, Rona, and the therapist worked on this part of their relationship life. During this process Rona could see how much her own original family experience had set her up to chase unrealistic expectations of her mother-in-law and to project much of what she had not worked out with her own mother and brother onto her marriage and the relationship with her mother-in-law. Richard could respond to his wife's diminished criticism of his mother by beginning the task of deidealizing her—something Rona had believed would never happen. This work produced a better than 25% improvement in Richard's symptoms, bringing the total improvement to 95% over 12 months.

As they prepared to wrap things up for a therapy vacation, a routine mammogram revealed that Rona had a suspicious lesion that turned out to be cancer of the breast. The therapist remembers wondering whether this misfortune represented a continuation of bad things happening around Richard or was just relationship reciprocity having its way. Another year of therapy followed Rona and Richard through her cancer treatment. Now, 5 years later, the therapist sees them occasionally around parenting issues with their adolescent sons. Richard has remained almost completely free of symptoms with occasional slips into dysthymic dreaming. Rona is free of any evidence of metastatic disease from her cancer. Rona and Richard are doing well together. A case that began as an individual with anxiety turned out to involve that individual's marriage and, in addition, the triangle with his mother.

Most clinicians have little difficulty seeing the relevance of family systems ideas, including triangles, in some contexts. These include the treatment of marital problems, problems between one or both parents and a child, and even symptoms in an individual child. However, when it comes to psychotherapy with individual adults, many therapists confine the application of systems ideas such as triangles mostly to exercises in the attainment of differentiation and autonomy.

In fact, there is a much broader use in individual work for these ideas and methods, especially the idea of triangles. Thinking about triangles can give the therapist a new set of treatment options when therapy with an individual is at an impasse. Dealing with the triangles surrounding an individual's problem can reinforce and consolidate the gains made from other work in psychotherapy and from the use of medication. In this chapter we show you how to look for and resolve triangles when you're working with a variety of individual patients.

Describing Anxiety

Most of the symptoms that present themselves as problems within an individual are manifestations of anxiety or depression, or a combination of both. The term *anxiety* has become too diffuse and generalized; it needs to be broken down into its component parts to be useful. Anxiety has biological and psychological elements, and patients experience anxiety subjectively in phenomenological and existential terms. Let's look at each of these elements of anxiety briefly.

Your heart stops and then takes off like a racehorse when a small airplane hits an air pocket. You suddenly become as alert as a hunted animal when you hear footsteps behind you on a dark city street. You feel a quick flash of fear when you're about to get an injection, but you can't think of anything to be afraid of. The great William James suggested long ago that feelings such as anxiety are an individual's conscious awareness of physiological reactions that precede a recognized emotion. Whether this is so or not has yet to be settled. Which comes first, the emotion or the physiological arousal, and what those physiological reactions are still is not certain. What is certain is that anxiety has many physiological manifestations. Some are specific to panic anxiety, others are peculiar to generalized anxiety, and some are present in both. They include palpitations, sweating, trembling or shaking, shortness of breath, chest pain or discomfort, nausea or abdominal distress, paresthesias, chills or hot flushes, muscle tension, and sleep disturbance.[3]

---

[3]American Psychiatric Association (1994, pp. 395, 436).

Psychological elements of anxiety are described in psychodynamic theories of the origin and symptoms of anxiety. According to Freudian drive theory, anxiety is a response to the feared consequences of acting on an unconscious wish. The wish is often aggressive, but it may be sexual. (You may remember feeling a surge of anxiety when you considered saying something really ugly to someone or when you stole a peek at something pornographic.) People who feel anxiety about the unconscious wish fear punishment should they act on that wish. The punishment they fear is related to what they learned to expect as a very young child. These punishments are the four great calamities of childhood: loss of the object (if I do something awful, Mommy will go away and leave me), loss of the object's love (Mommy and Daddy won't love me any more if I play with myself again), castration anxiety (most usefully understood as a symbol of severe and disabling punishment), and the condemnation of one's own superego (some things are so shameful that if we do them we become disgusted with ourselves). Because anxiety is so painful, we activate various defense mechanisms to keep us from acting on our impulses—thereby risking the dreaded consequences.

The self-psychological view of anxiety concerns the notion that those children who weren't adequately mirrored as children didn't learn to contain their emotions. Consequently, when something upsets them or even when they don't have an appreciative object mirroring self around, they're susceptible to uncontrollable upsurges of feeling—e.g., anxiety—from which they seek escape through some form of self-soothing ("pigging out" on Ben & Jerry's ice-cream) or excitement (snorting cocaine or watching X-rated videos).

Other common symptoms of anxiety described in DSM-IV include sensations of smothering, feeling of choking, derealization or depersonalization, fear of losing control or going crazy, fear of dying,[4] persistent fear of having additional attacks,[5] persistent thoughts, images, or impulses that people experience as intrusive,[6] restlessness, fatigue, difficulty concentrating or going blank, irritability.[7]

---

[4]American Psychiatric Association (1994, p. 395).

[5]American Psychiatric Association (1994, p. 402).

[6]American Psychiatric Association (1994, p. 422).

[7]American Psychiatric Association (1994, p. 436).

Most clinicians have also heard their patients describe their symptoms subjectively. These phenomenological descriptions of anxiety include a sense of apprehension, worry, a fear or dread without clear cause, a troubled state of mind about uncertain events, a sense of danger, lack of security, and a sense of impending doom. These feelings of anxiety seem to feed on themselves, to go beyond control, to become more real until anxiety becomes a way of life. Anxiety can show in relationships through overly positive statements, the tendency not to listen or to interrupt, excessive quantity or rapidity of speech, hyperactivity, impatience, and assuming that one knows the unknown. It may exist in the present, when panicky feelings of unknown origin limit movement, function, or ability to live in the moment. Mostly, these signs of anxiety suggest that anxiety may at bottom be people's attempt to control what they cannot control (others) or to avoid controlling what they can control (themselves).

Describing Depression

Depression can be very confusing. Its symptoms, like those of anxiety, are legion, but it can be useful to think about depression in biological, psychological, and phenomenological terms. Current thinking about the etiology of depression is predominantly biological. An insufficiency of the neurotransmitters serotonin, norepinephrine, or both, is thought to be the primary culprit in severe depression. (However, the life stress correlates of depression suggest that its etiology may be more complicated.) Biological symptoms of depression include sleep and appetite disturbances, psychomotor retardation or agitation, lack of energy, and loss of libido.[8]

Psychological views of depression usually implicate *loss* as the root of depression. The classical Freudian position is that, whereas anxiety is a signal that something awful might happen, depression is a signal that (unconsciously) something awful *has already* happened. So the loss in the present—say, the death of a beloved pet—triggers the (unconscious) belief that, because of one's own actions, one has lost something profound—one of the four calamities of childhood. "My cat is dead, and I'm lonely. Nobody really loves me. In fact, nobody has ever loved me. How could they, considering I'm such an angry, selfish person?" The self-psychological view deals with narcissistic

---

[8]American Psychiatric Association (1994, p. 327).

injury—loss of self-sustaining mirroring experiences—and the inability to control one's feelings.

Psychological symptoms include a depressed mood with feelings of sadness and emptiness or tearfulness, markedly diminished interest or pleasure in the activities of the day, feelings of worthlessness or excessive or inappropriate guilt, diminished ability to think or concentrate, recurrent thoughts of a death, suicidal ideation, or suicide attempt.[9]

Phenomenologically, patients with depressions may describe a state of uneasiness or potential distress about future uncertainties. They may go into the past in response to some stimulus that recalls bad memories. They describe withdrawal into self, lack of productivity, less contact with family and friends, introspection, and preoccupation with self. Anger may be a sign of underlying depression. Early in depression, there may be a desperate pursuit of others, but eventually, distance and withdrawal are present. Mood swings are common, and they include sadness, blueness, irritability, disinterest, lack of joy or enthusiasm, and varying periods of anxiety. Sufferers of depression sometimes report feelings of selfishness, worthlessness, and shame. They say they feel hopeless and helpless, and they believe that this state will always be. There is, deep inside, a penetrating feeling of emptiness and of being all alone.

Looking at Anxiety and Depression Combined

Most people appear in therapy with a mixture of symptoms of anxiety and depression. Usually one feeling predominates. This mixture includes, to varying degrees, a feeling of unsureness, being shaken, feeling insecure, and the sense that the ground under them is falling away. They often think that there is something undefined out there waiting for them, a sense of impending doom that does not disappear with reassurance from others. This varies daily with the depressed feelings of hopelessness and helplessness and the sense that this scenario will never go away. There is no light and no hope.

Every therapist at some time faces this multitude of symptoms and complaints. The complaint is familiar: either depression or anxiety. However, the meanings of these words are so diffuse and different that therapists must deal with each as an individual complaint. To

---

[9]American Psychiatric Association (1994, p. 327).

one person, depression means something that has taken over his life; to another, it means a "blueness" that will be gone after the first cup of coffee; to a third, it means a way of getting someone to sympathize with her and give her a hug. The same is true of anxiety. To one, it is the feeling before an exam that keeps the person at home studying; to another, it is a sense that the IRS will catch him in something he has done wrong; to a third, it is a sense of acute panic, of her impending death. Getting the patient to describe his or her experience is crucial. The description should include not only biological and psychological terms but also the way it seems to the patient.

To understand these symptoms, the therapist must ask questions about the specific complaint: When did it start? Where did it happen? Who was present and who was absent? What makes it better? What makes it worse? How did you deal with it? Who helped you and who did not? When did it go away? These and similar questions pin down the details and place the generic complaint of depression or anxiety in a context. The context gives specific meaning to the complaint. Depression and anxiety have different meanings depending on the context. There is no one universal definition of depression or anxiety. The symptoms are so variable that we must usually individualize the definition, though the general theme may be universal. Every anxiety, for example, is different from person to person in the story of its development. At the same time, it has the general characteristic of being a fear of loss of control over self or frustration at the impossibility of controlling others.

It is important for the therapist to be facile both with symptom checklists that document the presence or absence of anxiety and depression and to ask the kind of open-ended questions that engage the patient, allow for a contextualization of the symptoms, and limit therapist distortion.

PLACING INDIVIDUALS' SYMPTOMS IN CONTEXT

All symptoms are part of a context. The internal context includes a person's temperament, biological makeup, and psychological state. This last includes introjected good and bad objects from the past, and a person's feelings about these objects play out in the present with real representatives of the objects. These people are part of the external context. Triangles can make sense of this process. For example, a man plays out his ambivalent feelings about his mother in his relationship with his wife. A woman plays out her resentment at a dominating father in her dealings with a male supervisor. In traditional psychoanalysis, the patient plays out feelings about a parent (or another introjected object) with the analyst.

People who have been badly hurt by past experience may have decided to stay distant and disconnected from others to protect themselves from further hurt. They see the maximally distant, minimally involved position as the safe position. Their distance does protect them—but at the price of loneliness. These people develop symptoms "inside themselves." Perhaps they get depressed from loneliness or anxious when they have to relate to others (for example, at work). Whenever they engage others in relationships (twosomes), these are apt to become triangles when they run into problems. When relationships get too close for comfort, when people feel hurt or even that they *might* get hurt, they try to protect themselves. They may distance from the relationship, or they may try to stay in it by deflecting sore spots, actual or potential, into a triangle.

Triangles are kinds of defense mechanisms that are always present with depression and anxiety. The usual understanding of psychoanalytic theory is that people resort to defense mechanisms to control the ideas and impulses threatening to make them anxious or depressed. Defense mechanisms include repression, suppression, projection, denial, reaction formation, and the others that we learned in Psych 101. But in fact, anything can be used for defensive purposes—even apparently quite constructive activities. Not surprisingly, therefore, people even shift around in their relationships to defend themselves against experiencing painful feelings—and that's where triangles come in. Triangles may not be apparent immediately, but they will show eventually as the person with symptoms inside him- or herself begins to deal with those symptoms. Getting at all of them all the time is not necessary, however. As long as defenses work in an acceptable and workable way, and if their situation is tolerable inside and around themselves, people may decide that "tolerable" is as far as they wish to go. A man may handle his loneliness by a close association with his sister, and his wife may handle the resulting distance by developing a keen interest in art. This may be satisfactory to both and, in their view, not worth pursuing further. That triangle may work well until the sister dies, but it may fall apart when the man wants more closeness from his wife and asks her to give up her interest in art. Under stress, a potential triangle becomes not just active but clinically symptomatic.

We can manage the symptoms of anxiety and depression with medication, cognitive therapy, hypnosis, or strategic systems intervention to name just a few of the weapons at our disposal. In our experience, these methods are useful tools in symptom control and management. If the source of the anxiety and depression is acute or situational in nature, and therefore a time-limited one, symptom control may be all that a patient needs. In such cases, matching the intervention to the patient and her or his symptoms is sufficient. We do not intend to speak in derogatory terms about "mere" symptom control; in real life, most clinical practice in any health field is oriented to symptom control.

Paul Y., a 27-year-old carpenter, came for therapy complaining of anxiety. Paul was an only child whose father had left the family when Paul was 9. His mother sent him to live with her mother for 4 years while she tried to adjust to her husband's abandonment. Paul reported that she drank a lot, hung out in bars, and had affairs with many men during those years. When he was 13, his mother remarried and took Paul back. Over the next couple of years he heard the stories and found evidence of the dissipation of his mother's life during the previous 4 years.

When he was 14, Paul began to drink and use drugs. He also became sexually promiscuous, seeing girls and women as objects for his physical gratification and sources of validation for his attractiveness. He dropped out of high school at 16, and his alcohol abuse, drug abuse, and sexual promiscuity escalated. He had a son by one girlfriend. He couldn't hold a job and was always being fired for being late or not showing up at all.

Paul was referred by his mother, who was not aware of any specifics of his present complaint. He had asked her to find out from a nurse friend of hers the name of a good therapist. She did believe that he was immature and needed help. She had been worried about him since his adolescence because of what she saw as his poor adjustment to adult life. Paul thought she also had some guilt, thinking that maybe some of his problems were her fault.

At the time of presentation, he had a steady job, was helping to support his 5-year-old son, and regularly saw him. He denied current drug use but admitted to occasional heavy drinking on weekends ("I drink one or two dozen beers when I'm out with my friends"). Paul didn't currently have a girlfriend, but he was looking. He worried that he didn't feel closer to his son. He wished he could have the kind of relationship with him that he was always seeing on TV, where the father "takes the kid fishing and stuff," and where "the kid looks up to his father." He revealed that his father had begun writing to him occasionally about 2 years earlier, but Paul hadn't answered. He said that he got "really tense" even thinking about writing to his father. In fact, he told the therapist that just talking about it was making him nervous and sweaty at that very moment.

The therapist could not fully understand Paul's anxiety, it became evident, unless it was placed in the context of the triangles in which it was embedded. Here's why. His concerns focused on his relationship with his son and on his inability to form a long-term attachment with any of the women with whom he got involved. His attachment to his mother involved economic dependence, a powerful need for her approval, and a belief that she was wise and always right. This dependency and idealization colored his view of his son (a triangle) because he adopted her (his mother's) view of people whether he wanted to or not. In addition, his attachment to his mother put any woman he dated in the outside position in another triangle.

PAUL: Every time I start to feel close to a woman, I start to find some kind of fault.

THERAPIST: What sort of faults do you find? Is it different in each one, or is there some pattern?

PAUL: Well, with Madeline [his most recent girlfriend] I thought my mother wouldn't like her. Isn't that something? That was my first thought. I can't stand it.

THERAPIST: Is that your first thought about many of the women you've dated? That your mother wouldn't like them?

PAUL: Yeah. I'm too close to her, aren't I?

Paul's attachment to his mother needs to change in character if he is going to be able to form a long-term relationship with another woman. His attachment to his mother, and her influence over him, are related to his status as an only child in a one-parent family. He and his mother lived alone for years, during which his well-being was her only concern. During that time Paul had no contact at all with his father. In other words, his primary parental triangle had him and his mother in an overly close position, with his father in the outside position. Paul can work on establishing a relationship with his father, which will automatically shift the intensity of his closeness with his mother. It will create more of a balance in the primary parental triangle. Once his relationship with his mother is less intense, he should be freer to develop a closer relationship with a woman.

Paul's concern about his relationship with his son was tied to the same problem.

PAUL: When I'm with him, it's like I'm just putting in my time. I don't really feel close to him.

THERAPIST: Is it like the relationship between you and your father?

PAUL: I guess so. My mother refuses to have anything to do with Ronnie [his son]. She's never even seen him. I hate that. It makes me think there's something wrong with him.

THERAPIST: So, you feel distant from your son, your mother *is* distant from your son, and you and your mother are too close?

PAUL: Yeah. It's just like me and my mother and my father, huh?

Individuals most commonly come to treatment with symptoms driven by anxiety, depression, or both. Clinicians often define this as a process *only* inside the person. It's necessary, however, to see not only the intrapersonal process but also the systemic implications of the symptom. This means that the therapist treating an individual can move from the individual's internal states to the important dyad or dyads in his or her life, to the triangles in which he and or she the dyads are caught, and back again. Symptoms within an individual often mean that there are problems in relationships, and problems in relationships often mean that there are problems within an individual.

Alice H. came for a medication consult for phobic and depressive symptoms. She had been phobic since seventh grade, when she refused to go to school. Now she is reluctant to leave her house. It was when Alice was in the 7th grade that her father lost his job, the family had to move, and Alice's mother collapsed in her functioning. When she was 20, Alice married Vincent, an alcoholic truck driver who "straightened out" because of falling in love with her. After he got sober, Vincent became an overfunctioner. Alice's aunt had been her functional mother since her own mother's collapse. When her aunt died, Alice's grief disabled her, and she returned to having severe panic attacks and social phobia.

Surely there is intrapersonal process here. Perhaps because of her genetic inheritance from her mother, perhaps because of the traumatic events when she was in the 7th grade, Alice was "wired" for anxiety and depression. However, the systemic events (most recently her aunt's death, and her husband's overfunctioning) have pushed her beyond the point where her wiring can manage.

People try to keep internally and externally calm, safe, secure, and peaceful. When this is impossible in a world full of change, anxiety results. When one asks what is getting in the way of maintaining peace and safety, one begins to systematize a person's anxiety (that is, place it in the context of the family or other system of which the patient is a part). The same is true of depression. When a person gives up his or her attempts to control the environment, and realizes how limited he or she is in controlling anything but his or her own behavior, that person starts to feel helpless and hopeless. The question "Helpless and hopeless about what?" helps to place the individual's depression in context. The effort to maintain the peacefulness and serenity inside and around self is doomed to failure. The people around us with whom we connect always want the same thing, but on their terms, not necessarily ours. This produces a struggle for peacefulness and serenity, a struggle that is unavoidable because of the human desire to connect with others or to avoid them by distance.

When patients come in unhappy but not acutely symptomatic, most therapists immediately start asking what's going on in the person's life that might be causing the unhappiness. But when somebody comes in so acutely anxious that he or she can't sit still, entreats you—"Do something! I can't stand it. Can't you help me?"—most therapists get anxious themselves and think first of treating the symptoms, especially if they have easy access to medication. The same is true in cases of depression, especially if the patient mentions suicide. Therapists get so nervous, they ask all kinds of questions about suicide plans but never get around to saying, "You must feel awful. What's going on in your life?"

Anxiety is a manifestation of the threat to being safe. As anxiety builds, and the security operations fail, there is decreasing ability to distinguish a real threat (where anxiety is an appropriate response) from an imaginary one. Being anxious is appropriate if someone has a gun to your head; if you worry every time you go out that there might be someone around the corner who will put a gun to your head, that is a case of anxiety distorting reality. Biological correlates tie in with that. Constant anxiety depletes neurochemicals, feelings of helplessness due to loss of control set in, and depression takes over.

Therapeutic intervention can take place on one or several levels. One can intervene at the neurochemical level. One can also intervene on a cognitive level by trying to distinguish inappropriate anxiety from appropriate anxiety, or by analyzing the unsuccessful attempts to solve it, or by linking frustration to expectations and thereby systematizing the anxiety.

Depression is a loss, mostly of important objects, function, or status, but studies point to a correlation between systemic stress and what psychiatry has called endogenous depression. The sense of loss is an internal emotional reaction to events in a person's life. Such events can produce (1) shifts in relationship needs, (2) stress or demands on a relationship, (3) unmet or unreasonable expectations, (4) silent or overt relationship conflict. For example, Joe P. was a 50-year-old man retired on disability from his law practice because of chronic lymphoma. His inability to work produced a loss of focus for his day and an experience of uselessness. He felt that his life was over and that never again would anyone respect him for his intelligence and litigation skills. These narcissistic supplies obtained at work had contributed substantially to his sense of well-being. Their loss had created a developmental challenge of sorts—not only must he now struggle with his fear of dying, but he must also turn to connecting with his family in a different way. Thus he would regain some of the lost supplies and the support he needed to adjust his life and deal with his lymphoma. The transition was difficult at best. "Iron Joe" tried to be strong, but the internal manifestations of his loss made him irritable toward and critical of his wife and daughter. His wife and daughter in turn pulled together in a kind of alliance to avoid his criticism and irritation. Now Joe was on the outside of a triangle. This position in the triangle reinforced his negative emotional state, which raised his level of irritability and criticism, and so on.

When you consider systemic stress, you place the symptom in the context of a system. When you systematize, if triangles are there, they will become clear.

Being caught in a triangle and unable to free oneself is the most frustrating feeling in the world. Stress, anxiety, depression, and triangulation—all this is tied in to the ongoing fear of incorporation or abandonment. People are trying to find a balance, which is impossible, and they never get to it. That failure can create the anxiety and depression.

INDICATIONS FOR WORK WITH TRIANGLES IN INDIVIDUAL THERAPY

There are at least three sets of circumstances in clinical work with individuals where a working knowledge of relationship triangles is important, if not essential. Such circumstances usually present in a mix, but with one more prominent than the other two. Any one of them is a red flag that suggests the need to think about triangles. They are relationship problems, developmental difficulties, and refractory psychiatric symptoms.

1. The individual presents complaining of a *relationship problem* that is firmly embedded in a triangle of which the parties are unaware. Catherine C., a large woman by anyone's standards, carried herself with grace and charm. She smiled easily and was a natural at putting other people at ease in her presence. Most folks warmed to her quickly and found her easier than most to talk to, especially about personal things. These natural skills had helped to foster a highly successful career as a psychiatric social worker. Catherine was nationally prominent in several professional organizations and had a large network of people she considered friends. At age 40 she had already mourned the probable loss of reproductive function, but she still had hope for being married someday.

Catherine was no stranger to psychotherapy, having been in therapy early in her career as part of her professional development. None of her therapy had solved the problem of her life's major nemesis, her mother. For many years Catherine had felt a sense of mastery over the relationship. Professional accomplishment and the frenetic activity associated with it had justified a certain distance between them. Catherine had abandoned the relationship field to her younger sister, who, in spite of much less accomplishment, had always basked in their mother's praise. In some ways, this specialness of her sister Mary had been a source of relief to Catherine. Since their father had died 5 years earlier, Mary had pretty much taken over responsibility for their mother's well-being. Catherine and Mary would chat weekly by telephone, and once a month Catherine would visit to see her beloved niece and nephew. She would talk to her mother a couple of times a month, and more months than not they would get together for dinner.

The news of her mother's cancer had somehow changed all that. It had awakened in Catherine a longing for a connection with her mother that she thought she had left behind. In the 6 months since the diagnosis of her mother's terminal pancreatic cancer, Catherine had attempted to bridge the distance between them. She wanted to give the relationship one last try and her mother one last chance to be the mother Catherine needed. It wasn't working. Catherine left the time spent with her mother feeling empty and hopeless about the relationship. This is not to mention the anger bordering on rage she felt when her mother would use their time together to rave about Mary as a wife and mother and about the wonders of grandchildren.

A few days before coming for a consultation, Catherine had surprised herself by bursting into tears as she left the hospital. Catherine told the therapist about walking down Main Street, tears streaming down her face, wishing intensely that her father was still alive.

Catherine was a successful woman with considerable psycho-logical savvy. She was a good candidate for *coaching*. The therapist tracked with her how her relationship with her mother worked. What were the triggers that set Catherine off? How did the triangles in which the relationship with her mother was embedded work? Once these processes were clear, the therapist and Catherine worked out experiments for changing them. Catherine tried them out and brought the results into therapy for clarification and modification.

If Catherine had been a different kind of person, coaching might not have been appropriate. If she had been less high-functioning and more anxious, *direct intervention* might have been indicated. This would mean bringing other members of Catherine's relationship system into therapy and working with the main triangles directly. For instance, the therapist might have asked Catherine to bring her sister to one or more sessions. In those sessions, they might have explored their history with each other, with their mother, and with their father.

A significant part of Catherine's loss and frustration, both of which fed her symptoms, was tied to her relationship with her mother and the triangle with her mother and sister. Because Catherine wasn't her sister, she couldn't have the same kind of relationship with her mother that her sister had. Trying to have what she could not have complicated her relationship with both her mother and her sister. Not integrating her specialness to her father as a factor in her mother's criticism missed an important "interlocking triangle" in this clinical scenario. Simply by asking a question such as "How did your parents come to divide the two of you up like this?" can begin the process of integration.

If these triangles weren't dealt with in Catherine's treatment, we could assume the following outcomes. Mother would go to her grave too negative about Catherine and too positive about her sister. Catherine would continue to experience loss and frustration about her inability to have a relationship with her mother, and that loss and frustration would carry over into her relationship with her sister. The sisters would play out in their relationship whatever the underlying conflict was between their parents. Catherine would become a likely candidate for a chronic depression that would respond only partially to medication.

Whether through coaching or direct intervention, working the triangles put Catherine's feelings into a context. Helping her to define and work the key triangles that fed her symptoms markedly enhanced symptom relief. It also enabled her to attain a developmentally appropriate relationship with her sister as they dealt with the death of their mother and with the rest of their lives as surviving family members.

In therapy, working the triangles also avoids two dangerous traps. One is the trap of being too "supportive" of Catherine and reinforcing her sense of entitlement to her reactive feelings.

The other trap is losing sight of the fact that, for Catherine, having a functional relationship with her mother does *not* mean making nice-nice with her mother without changing anything. It says to Catherine, "You're caught up in a *process* that has you stuck. You, as well as your mother and sister, are involved in that process. To get unstuck, you must find out how the whole process works and then change your part in it."

In addition, Catherine's tearfulness can be the focal point for evaluating whether she is clinically depressed.

THERAPIST: What's your sleeping pattern been like since your mother got sick?

CATHERINE: I have trouble falling asleep some nights, but I wake up a couple of times during the night every night.

2. Some individuals present with *developmental difficulties,* such as an inability to leave home or form an attachment that will lead to marriage, that have been refractory to other forms of treatment. This is another indication that work with triangles is going to be important. Rod T. was a single, 38-year-old bond trader on Wall Street: successful, handsome, intelligent, and articulate. He was athletically

built, 6½ feet tall, and invariably came to sessions in his green Jaguar, wearing running shorts and a cut-off T-shirt (his appointments were always on Saturday morning). He came for evaluation after the breakup of a 4-year relationship with a woman whom he fully intended to marry. The reason he gave for the breakup was that he couldn't deal with her 8-year-old son by a previous marriage. He complained of lack of energy, no enjoyment in running and playing squash, intermittent tearfulness, and early morning wakening. These symptoms had been plaguing him for 6 months.

The use of Prozac or some similar medication might have helped the symptoms of Rod's chronic low-grade depression, although Rod refused to take anything. "I really don't believe in taking drugs that alter my mind." Whether he took medication or not, how he dealt with an abundance of interlocking triangles from his past and present relationships would be key to his internal emotional state and to his relationship life.

The genogram revealed some important history. Rod's older brother and only sibling had been killed in an auto accident at age 24, leaving behind a wife and two children. Rod had been 18 at the time, and his brother was very important to him. Six years later, Rod's mother had died of a "broken heart." Rod described her as having never been the same after her older son's death. Rod's first engagement was broken 6 months after his mother's sudden death. He continued to have an active relationship with his sister-in-law, his nieces, and their stepfather.

It turned out that Rod was developmentally frozen at age 18, when his "superstar" idealized brother had been killed, his mother had become dysfunctional, and he had become the caretaker of his competent but "negative and critical" father. The therapist approached these triangles in the first session.

THERAPIST: How would your life be different if your brother and mother hadn't died?

ROD: Totally different.

THERAPIST: How?

ROD: Then I'd have someone to approve of the choices I make in relationships and to encourage me to go on and take the risk.

This exchange offered an encouraging opening to the therapist to explore with Rod the connection he had now made between the loss of his brother and mother and his difficulty in freeing himself from his father and forming a new primary relationship. The exchange meant that he was willing to work on the unresolved problems there rather than insisting on some dating tips and advice on how to deal with women. Underneath his bluster and his need to let the therapist know how smart and successful he was, there was a willingness to listen, learn, and try something new.

3. The individual presents with *psychiatric symptoms* such as depression or anxiety that have been *refractory* to medication and previous attempts at psychotherapy. The patient complains of these symptoms and their implications without an explicit reference to any relationship. In these cases, there's a need to review the medications that have been tried, the results (or lack of) that have been obtained, and any side effects. The patient's symptoms then need to be placed in the context of his or her family, occupational life, and previous therapists, in search of the triangles that may be the obstacles to the patient's recovery.

Greg D. was a 52-year-old widower. He was a middle manager in an avionics plant, and his wife had died 2 years previously after a long bout with breast cancer. The physician who had referred Greg was puzzled by a mediocre response, first to Paxil and then to Prozac. He thought that perhaps Greg's children were in some way keeping his guilt alive. Greg complained of early morning wakening, constant fatigue, hopelessness, feelings of intense guilt about his wife's death, frequent somatic symptoms, and anxiety about dying himself. He said that these symptoms had persisted unchanged for almost the entire time since his wife died. Prozac had produced between 35% and 40% improvement.

First, the therapist encouraged Greg to continue his antidepressants and asked permission to speak with the prescribing physician. Greg agreed willingly. Second, the therapist tried to contextualize the symptoms to better understand Greg's depression and its nonresponsiveness to treatment. He started by exploring Greg's relationship with his late wife and with his children. This led to Greg's revealing a 10-year extramarital affair. He had profound guilt and was unable to talk about it with anyone except his lover, whom in some strange way he held responsible for his wife's death. The key triangles were now on the table. Once they were, and once Greg had begun to work on detriangling himself, the logjam in Greg's treatment came unstuck.

Just as it is a clinical fact that anxiety and depression are also linked to neurohormonal changes at the neurosynapse, we have tried to show from our clinical experience that the origination and treatment of anxiety and depression are also linked to relationship triangles in the affected individual's life. A working knowledge of relationship triangles is an important added tool in the clinical management of anxiety and depression in individuals. The next chapter contains a further elaboration of the use of coaching and direct intervention with triangles in individual therapy.

CHAPTER EIGHT

Coaching and Direct Intervention with Triangles in Individual Therapy

In the last chapter we established that individual cases are most likely to benefit from triangle therapy when they present in one of three ways—as relationship problems, as developmental difficulties, or as problems refractory to other methods of intervention. We also proposed that the clinical interventions used in these cases can be either *coaching* or *direct intervention*. Coaching an individual to do triangle work in his or her family or work system is more effective with people who are functioning at a high level. These people can step somewhat outside the ongoing emotional process, slow down their own emotional reactivity, figure out the structure of a particular relationship set and how the emotional process flows, and form an experimental plan of action. Direct intervention, by which we mean bringing one or more of the triangle members into therapy and working with the triangle there, is better suited for those who aren't able to detach themselves from the problem sufficiently. They remain reactive and caught up in the emotional process in a way that blinds them to options for dealing with it. It takes direct intervention to depolarize the conflict, decrease the heat, and bring light to bear on the situation.

The cases that follow are meant to give you a fuller sense of how to do triangle therapy with individuals when their problems fit into one of the three categories of relationship problems, developmental difficulties, or problems refractory to other methods of intervention.

CASES THAT PRESENT
WITH RELATIONSHIP PROBLEMS

Jeanne's Problem—Business or Personal?

Jeanne Y. was a 50-year-old investment counselor—attractive, intelligent, and looking 10 years younger than her stated age. She came to therapy following a crisis at work. Until the crisis, she had enjoyed a good working relationship with her superiors, her colleagues, and her clients. Economic conditions changed, however, and the company's clients were buying fewer of certain derivative products in which she specialized. Trying to recoup some of their losses, Jeanne's boss led an effort to develop and market a new investment product without fully disclosing the significant risks inherent in the product. One of Jeanne's best clients discovered this on his own, and brought the matter to Jeanne's attention.

Besides having some ethical concerns about the lack of disclosure, Jeanne felt caught between loyalty to her boss and obligations to her client. Her boss tried to gloss over the problem and minimize the ethical issues. Jeanne demanded full disclosure to the few clients who had already bought the product and a willingness by the company to buy it back from those who wanted out when informed of the risk. Jeanne's ethically-driven behavior allied her with her client. Her boss was in the outsider position, angry but reluctant to dismiss Jeanne or to write off the client. Jeanne's position had been based on her ethical principles, but she was unable to control her anxiety when faced with her boss's accusations of disloyalty. So she came to therapy.

Jeanne's therapist coached her to try to neutralize this triangle by holding her "I-position" based on her ethical principles and be ready to deal with the fallout from both her boss and her client. As she worked on this task, Jeanne began to realize how much she had fostered the client's dependence on her. She had spent excessive amounts of time listening to his personal problems and had made light of his infrequent sexual innuendoes, all with the goal of keeping his business. It was as if she didn't have enough confidence in her talents as an investment adviser and needed these other perks to satisfy the client. Her boss's response to the crisis highlighted for Jeanne the many times he had failed to include her in important meetings or to inform her about policies and plans. She realized that her boss valued her charm and sales ability but undervalued her creativity, intelligence, and good judgment.

As Jeanne progressed in therapy and in her work on the business triangle, she felt empowered and no longer trapped at work. She eventually changed jobs and started to reflect on the meaning of all she had been doing for her personal relationships. As she did this, she began to see just how clinging and dependent her husband had become, and how she had fostered that. She even allowed herself to remember how her 80-year-old father had for years used her for investment tips while excluding her from estate-planning meetings with her three brothers. Jeanne defined her relationships with her husband and her father as her next triangular challenge.

Lucie—A Single Mother and Her Only Son

Lucie V. was 36 when she came for therapy. She was concerned about her 19-year-old son, Ben, her only child. He was away at college and would often call her late at night, anxious and worried about his studies. He'd begin by saying that he couldn't sleep and was having fantasies that when he was through with school he wouldn't be able to survive on his own—that he wouldn't find a job, know how to fill out tax returns, find a mechanic for his car. Then he'd say that he had a test the next day and hadn't studied for it.

Lucie was a single parent and was upset about Ben being so anxious. She wanted to find a way to make him go to therapy. Instead, she told him that everything would be fine, and then she'd give him advice about organizing his time so that he could study more effectively. Lucie wondered why she behaved this way with her son and decided it was somehow linked with her guilt about divorcing his father. Ben's father was uninvolved with him except financially, and Lucie also wanted to find a way to convince him to take more interest in their son. This is a description, of course, of an overfunctioner caught in a triangle with her ex-husband and her son. She was trying to fix her son and his relationship with his father, something she'd been doing for years.

The therapist began by trying to get Lucie to experiment with drawing some boundaries—giving less advice to Ben and asking him not to call after 10:30 P.M. unless it was an emergency. While conducting the experiment, she was to monitor her emotional state and to observe any changes in her relationship with Ben. She hoped he might call his father to complain about her. To help Lucie distance herself from her son, the therapist linked the therapy process to her extended family by asking her how her life would have been different if, like Ben, she'd been an only child.

Lucie began to focus on the triangle involving herself, her mother, and her older sister, Carla. Mother would call Lucie with complaints about Carla. "Carla never called." "Carla was wasting her money by buying a car that was too expensive." "Carla would never find a man if she didn't stop being so nasty to everyone." Lucie, having her own negative history with her sister, would join her mother in bad mouthing Carla. Carla was 6 years older than Lucie, and they had been very close when they were children. Lucie remembered them playing school (Carla always played the teacher) and talking about all kinds of things. All that changed when Carla left for college and escaped from her conflicted relationship with her mother. Lucie felt abandoned. She realized that with her father's recent death and her mother's failing health, Carla was the only family she would have. It made sense to her to do some work on altering her reactivity with her sister and on getting out from between her mother and her sister.

To accomplish that goal, Lucie set up a series of monthly dinner engagements with Carla. She told her sister how lonely she was without Ben at home and how much she now needed the big sister who'd been there when they were little. Carla responded positively, and movement in the triangle began to shift.

Lucie's therapist also focused on the triangles that fed the problems with Ben. If she could help Lucie decrease her anxiety, she'd transmit less of it to Ben, she'd bail him out less, make fewer excuses for him, and his functioning might improve.

CASES WITH DEVELOPMENTAL PROBLEMS

Joshua—A Young Man Back at Home

Joshua F. was a 26-year-old single man living with his parents. He had moved out after college and had gotten a job as a bank auditor in Virginia. While living in Virginia he had been seriously hurt in an automobile accident, and he had come home to recuperate. He had moved out again but returned after several months. He came for therapy at his parents' insistence. They thought it was time for Joshua to move out permanently and be on his own, and Joshua agreed with them. He felt frustrated and angry with himself that he just couldn't face being on his own again, and he was angry with his parents, especially his father, for pushing him.

This inability to move out after he had recuperated strongly suggested a developmental problem that was complicated by (not caused by) his accident. It was as if Joshua had barely gotten out the first time, and after the accident he got mired in his primary parental triangle. In the aftermath of his accident, Joshua had developed symptoms of depression, seasoned with episodes of intense anxiety. During these episodes, he'd fluctuate back and forth between his fears of leaving home and feeling trapped there forever.

Joshua had always been caught in the middle between his parents. His present situation, the depression and anxiety, and his low functioning were complicated by the accident, his physical pain, and his drawn-out lawsuit seeking financial compensation for his loss of functioning and suffering. In the background, however, was perhaps the most important factor in his situation, predating his accident—his position in his primary parental triangle. During the therapist's investigation of Joshua's past and present relationship with his parents, she learned that early in Joshua's life his mother had been the beneficiary of a large trust fund from her grandparents. She had given Joshua's father considerable amounts of money to start up several business ventures, all of which had failed. Joshua's most vivid memories of his father were of him leaving to play golf four or five mornings a week. He remembered his father not coming home much, and when he did, he'd drink too much and criticize Joshua on the occasions when he spoke to him. Joshua didn't remember his parents ever discussing any of these issues. Mrs. F. never spoke to her husband about how she felt about his business failures His parents were quite distant and appeared to live parallel lives. Mrs. F. regularly commiserated with Joshua about his father's criticisms of him, and she managed to convey to Joshua her disrespect for his father's unproductive life style. The therapist suggested to Joshua that it might be useful to include his parents in therapy for a few sessions.

In the conjoint sessions, the therapist began by reviewing the parents' concerns about Joshua—was his pain real, was he getting adequate care from a pain clinic, and was he becoming addicted to pain medication? After listening to their anxieties and discussing them, the therapist then broached the subject of Joshua's living at home and the difficulty he was having in leaving. She asked Mr. and Mrs. F. if they had thought about how they could be supportive of their son without being enabling. This discussion led to two suggestions from the therapist aimed at changing the structure of the primary parental triangle.

First, the therapist talked with Mrs. F. about how helpful it would be if she could learn not to pump her anxiety into Joshua. She pointed out that Mrs. F. could instead come in and talk to the therapist about things that were bothering her, or talk to her husband or family or a friend. But she should avoid making Joshua her confidante.

Second, Mrs. F. needed to discuss clearly with Joshua how financially supportive she was willing to be. Her wealth made it possible for her to arrange that Joshua would never have to work again, but that might be more damaging than helpful. The therapist suggested that perhaps Joshua and his mother might negotiate the issue: Joshua could begin by telling her what he needed in the way of financial support, and Mrs. F. could evaluate whether she thought doing that would be supportive or enabling. The therapist offered to help in that negotiation if it turned out to be necessary.

Third, the therapist talked with Mr. F. about his job in this family experiment. He could view Joshua's misfortune as an opportunity to do what he had never done—build a relationship with Joshua. Mr. F.'s only way of relating to Joshua during his childhood and college years had been to criticize him. Now was his chance to develop a personal connection with his adult son. The therapist suggested that Joshua and his father spend relationship time together, doing something they both enjoyed. She also thought it might be interesting for the two of them to get together and talk about Mr. F.'s father and in general about the men in the family—how well or poorly they did, and why.

During this work, Joshua, albeit with substantial apprehension, found an apartment in the same town, moved out of his parents' home, and found a job as a loan officer in a local bank. At this point, the family decided to take a vacation from therapy. In her last session with Joshua, the therapist asked him if he thought his mother would ever take the therapist up on her offer to come in and talk about what bothered her. That question caused Joshua to raise the issue of his parents' marriage. He told the therapist that during his most recent dinner date with his father, Joshua had asked him how he'd evaluate his marriage. Joshua told his father that he'd started thinking about getting married some day, and was curious about how his father viewed marriage in general and his marriage in particular. His father had changed the subject. Clearly, therapy with this family had miles to go.

Compelling circumstances that affect an individual, such as a serious accident, often lead clients and therapists to overlook the family context, as if problems are either in the individual or in the surrounding relationship system. Human beings tend to think in all-or-nothing, either–or terms. Integrating the individual and the system regularly turns out to be harder than it sounds. Although most people accept the importance of integrating nature and nurture, shaping experience and DNA, they still behave as if everything important happens either at the neurosynapse or at the mother's knee.

Joshua's accident and the physical and emotional aftermath adversely affected him and everyone who had a relationship with him. The therapist hoped that the direct intervention with his parents would foster continued efforts to move Joshua and his family toward better functioning and improved connection with one another. His strengths and flaws as an individual, and those of his relationship system, are important in accomplishing these goals.

Cynthia—A Middle-Aged Nurse at Work and at Home

Cynthia U. called in an agitated state, explaining that she had been crying, depressed, and without sleep for 2 days following an intense confrontation with her boss. She felt frightened and out of control, and she had asked a physician with whom she was friendly for a referral. Cynthia was a head nurse who had "lost it" with her supervisor when that supervisor informed her that she was reassigning Cynthia to another floor the following month. Cynthia had been happy working in pediatrics, and the supervisor wanted her to move to Ob–Gyn. At 48 and after 26 years with an exemplary record of nursing, Cynthia felt abused and said so, loudly. Cynthia was perplexed by her reaction, since refusing an assignment, let alone having a public outburst, was totally uncharacteristic of her. She had been unable to return to the hospital since the incident, and she was having difficulty pulling herself together.

Like most people approaching 50, Cynthia was under considerable pressure. The past year had been particularly stressful. Eight months before the encounter with her supervisor, she had begun hormone replacement therapy and had had a hysterectomy, neither of which had resolved her physical problems. She believed that her hormone levels were now even more unbalanced than when she'd started the treatment, contributing to her uncharacteristic emotionality. In addition, Cynthia's older son left for college that fall, and she worried a lot about how he would adjust.

Other pressures were related to both her husband's and her own extended families. Cynthia grew up in an Italian American family. She was the oldest of three children, having a younger brother and a sister. Her parents, who were retired and sickly, were her major concern. Cynthia's sister had been married to a man whom Cynthia described as crazy. In the latest crisis, Cynthia's sister had called to report that her husband had tried to set fire to their house and that she had called the police. In the aftermath of that incident, the sister and her three children had moved in with Cynthia's parents.

Cynthia's parents and brother (who lived out of state) called her daily, sometimes more often, to complain about the situation. She was frantic about her parents' physical and emotional well-being. She was also angry with all her family members because they refused to take her advice.

Cynthia's role in the family had always been that of the overly responsible caretaker. She was the one the rest of the family came to to solve problems and express unhappiness about others. She had been the one who behaved, always complying with her parents' wishes even though she felt they ignored her and didn't value her as much as they did her younger siblings. She was never pretty like her sister or brilliant like her brother. She described her relationship with her mother over the years as difficult. Although her mother called her with all her problems, she became angry with Cynthia if Cynthia suggested solutions. Cynthia's dad was a quiet, passive man, reluctant to express his opinion. More recently, with the deterioration of his health, Cynthia feared that the increased stress from having her sister and her sister's children move in would kill him.

In her husband's family, Cynthia found the approval and attention she'd always longed for. Cynthia and her mother-in-law were like sisters and spoke every day, at least on the phone. In the previous year, after an unsuccessful intervention with Cynthia's husband's alcoholic brother, Cynthia's relationship with her mother-in-law changed. It had been a relationship in which Cynthia had felt nurtured, but now Cynthia's mother-in-law began calling Cynthia with her anxiety over the treatment failure of her alcoholic son. This shifted the relationship, and further drained Cynthia's energy—in a place where nurturing and support had been for years. Cynthia couldn't take it and had been trying to avoid her.

Cynthia came to therapy with a litany of symptoms. She had no energy, but although she always felt tired, she had difficulty staying asleep at night, waking up two or more times every night. She looked to herself like her old and haggard mother, instead of the vital woman she used to be. She was irritable and had experienced an increase in the frequency of aches and pains in her head and back. She had been having palpitations. In short, she had a pervasive listlessness and negativity familiar to many of us in our middle years. Feeling this way made it difficult for her to work, a major area of competency for her for years.

By assessing the stressors in Cynthia's life using a genogram, the therapist could see certain things much more clearly. First, changes that are common in midlife had bombarded Cynthia in the previous year. Illness, the threatened change in her job, her son's leaving for school, and the loss of the comfort of her mother-in-law had all contributed to rising anxiety in the family and in Cynthia. Second, Cynthia was an overresponsible and serious woman, and her response to stress was to try harder to fix things in everyone's life. When she couldn't, she became angry and felt guilty. She then tried harder and reached a state of burnout. By the time her superior informed her of her job reassignment, she had no emotional reserves left.

Whatever approach a therapist might take to treat Cynthia's emotional turmoil—behavioral, psychodynamic, family systems, cognitive—addressing her behavior in her extended family triangles, especially the primary parental triangle, is crucial in helping Cynthia return to functioning. A return to functioning first meant getting back to work. The therapist addressed Cynthia's individual functioning by reframing her situation. This involved coaching her on how to make a cognitive shift, altering her overly negative perspective, and acquiring a more positive view to facilitate the kind of changes that were going to be necessary. It also involved helping her see that she had more going on in her life than a job change and a problem with her boss. This shift helped Cynthia to see that in reality she had a long-term, good relationship with her boss, and that his shifting her assignment was a vote of confidence in her abilities rather than a criticism. The therapist normalized Cynthia's difficulty around midlife anxieties and pressures, and the tough situations she was dealing with, by reviewing with her how predictable many of them were and how understandable her response was. This made it easier for Cynthia to develop a rationale for having "lost it" at work: her overresponsible and serious nature, the year of physical and emotional change, her inability ever to walk away from a problem, and her need to ease up.

Speaking to the triangles in her life might also prevent a recycling of this scenario should Cynthia's level of stress increase due to another midlife mishap. As an adult, Cynthia's way of relating to her parents had been to continue her overly responsible role in the family. She was still her mother's ear, but not her mother's favorite; that was a role reserved for her baby sister. Her relationship with her father, more distant than ever as he developed Parkinson's disease, became increasingly less rewarding. Cynthia's position with both parents was one-dimensional, a relationship without options. Cynthia was caught in a pattern of being the problem-solver with her entire extended family, not free to operate on a person-to-person basis with any one of them. Being stuck in this place left her without a "real" relationship with her parents at a time in her life when she was surrounded by loss or potential loss. Her contact with her family left her angry, frustrated, and frightened. In a way, the senior nursing supervisor had been a parental figure in her life, one she felt had approved of her until their recent confrontation.

The therapist assessed Cynthia's extended family and in-law triangles. Cynthia made no secret of the impact that the shift in her previously supportive and close relationship with her mother-in-law had had on her. It was clear to the therapist that the soil had been fertile for Cynthia's connection to her husband's mother, because she was a warm and nurturing woman who was excited about having a "daughter" like Cynthia; this was a sharp contrast with Cynthia's perception of her own mother. Losing her mother-in-law's support and nurturing hurt.

Underpinning her need for her mother-in-law were the difficult relationships Cynthia had in her own extended family. Over the years she had handled her disappointment in her relationships with her mother and father with distance and ritualized contact. She maintained her polite, goody two-shoes operating style for all the years until her sister's difficult marital situation caused a change in the way the family operated. Cynthia became the person everyone turned to to resolve what had become an unresolvable situation. She was caught between her own reactivity and her family, and had real anxiety and fears over everyone's safety.

When the therapist discussed with Cynthia her role with her in-laws, it became clear that Cynthia was overfunctioning in that family, too. Her husband had thrown up his hands when it came to his alcoholic brother. He had no patience for his mother's infantilizing him. He also felt frustrated that Cynthia had been in the middle between his mother and him, pressuring him to do something so that his mother would not be upset. The therapist coached Cynthia to turn her husband's family problems back over to her husband and just have a woman-to-woman relationship with her mother-in-law. Cynthia liked the idea, although she admitted it would be difficult work. The therapist made a mental note that the change in this in-law triangle might unearth some conflict between Cynthia and her husband.

Addressing Cynthia's primary parental triangle was crucial to her recovery from her depression. The therapist employed the following strategy to alter Cynthia's position in the triangle with her parents. First, Cynthia was coached to stop trying to resolve her sister's and parents' living situation. This meant teaching Cynthia how to behave in a less parental and more helpless way. She admitted to her mother that she was at a loss. She said that the problem was tough and that it saddened her that she was failing the family, especially her mother. This was a totally new and nondefensive position for Cynthia, and initially it made her quite anxious and worried. However, when she realized that nothing awful happened as a result, she was greatly relieved.

Next, the therapist coached Cynthia to narrow the distance between her sick father and herself. She was to do that by making 1- or 2-hour, one-on-one visits with him in which she just "hung out" and didn't discuss family problems. If they did talk, Cynthia would ask her father to talk about his past, perhaps about his parents. She was coached to monitor her mother's reaction to this shift and to make sure she brought her mother a little gift when she came to visit or spend some time alone with her. Cynthia planned her visits when her sister wasn't around, as it would have overloaded Cynthia to also have to deal with her sister. That would come later.

The frequency of sessions had been about once a month. The therapist raised with Cynthia the possibility of bringing in her whole family for some direct intervention, but they all had their own versions of therapy allergy. Cynthia thought it wouldn't work.

Her position in her primary parental triangle had changed over time. As in all triangles, the relationships and the intensity of the reactivity between people vary from day to day and from issue to issue. When you're addressing a clinical problem that involves a triangle such as Cynthia's, it isn't helpful to focus on the parents' motivation, or even their fault, in the triangle. It's important to remember that everyone in a triangle plays a part. To be successful in coaching a patient to change his or her position, both the therapist's and the patient's reactivity need to be under control. The fact that Cynthia was the unsung hero in her family may have contributed to her feeling victimized and helpless to change her position. The therapist needed to be clear that Cynthia was becoming a hero to herself with the new ways she was operating in the key triangles of her life.

Cynthia was a better coaching subject than the therapist had predicted—she was highly motivated to regain some control of her life and these methods made a lot of sense to her. Today she is much less tired out and has even had some decent talks with her mother about missing her son.

CASES OF REFRACTORY ANXIETY OR DEPRESSION

Denise—A Stubborn Depression with Somatic Complaints

Denise T. loved the juggling act that was her life. She was a mortgage loan officer for a large financial institution, a married mother of two, and 45 years old. All her life she had amazed the people who knew her with her energy and ease of accomplishment. Approximately a year before coming to therapy she began to experience incapacitating headaches, preceded by nausea, photophobia, and other visual symptoms. In the beginning, she had had the headaches only about once a month, but recently she was losing up to 6 days a month of work because of them. When the pain came, she had no choice but to retreat to her darkened bedroom, take her pain medicine, and sleep until it was over.

Her internist and a consulting neurologist had tried their best to bring her relief, and when they met with only limited success, they referred Denise to the headache clinic of a major teaching hospital in New York City. At the headache clinic, the doctor in charge created what he called his special individualized headache cocktail, consisting of a combination of anti-inflammatory agents, muscle relaxants, and tricyclic antidepressant medication. This regimen brought her some relief in the headaches' intensity. The neurologist also recommended psychotherapy for what he saw as her accompanying depression.

When she came for psychotherapy, she hoped that both the intensity and frequency of her headaches would decrease in time. She was less concerned about depression than about her headaches. The initial evaluation in therapy revealed substantial stressors and challenges in Denise's life over the past 18 months: (1) Her father had died after a 6-month battle with pancreatic cancer; (2) her mother had put the family home on the market and moved in with Denise; (3) her husband had taken a new job in a city 200 miles away and was only home on weekends; (4) her youngest child and only son had left for college. The implications of these events for Denise's emotional life were profound. First, she had lost the connection with her father and the emotional support and unconditional approval she had always received from him. Second, she was now subject to constant "constructive criticism" from her mother, which she used to receive only once a week on the telephone. Third, her husband returned home every weekend and gave her his version of constructive criticism. Finally, her son's departure had robbed her of his reassuring presence and had created an emotional void in her life.

Besides all that, her husband's attitude toward her headaches implied that they were psychosomatic (which to him meant a figment of her overactive imagination) and that she was using them to punish him for taking the job in another city. In fact, Denise did think that it was a strange coincidence that Dan's new job opportunity had arisen shortly after her mother had moved in. She acknowledged that she was angry with him, but she knew that her pounding pain was very real. When the therapist asked how she thought her anger at Dan came out, Denise described difficulty sleeping, overeating, and her inability to think about anything else.

Most clinical situations represent a triangle waiting to happen (or, more likely, a triangle that has already happened and is waiting to make an appearance). The symptom bearer often feels victimized or misunderstood by family members or health care professionals. The tightrope the clinician must walk is to provide the necessary validation, empathy, and support without joining in on blaming the family or avoiding contact with them, and without becoming an advocate for the patient with his or her family. Being able to see triangles and manage them is critical to walking this tightrope successfully. Walking the tightrope gives the patient support and calms down the family, enabling them to be less reactive and therefore more supportive themselves.

The theory here is that Denise's losses, combined with the developmental and structural changes in the family, had set off a biological vulnerability to headaches. They had also activated the dysfunctional adult triangle (her mother and her husband both trying to fix her). Denise had distanced herself from their criticism by moving toward neurologists for her headaches and toward psychiatrists for her depression. Introducing myriad physicians had created therapy triangles, as the physicians had aligned themselves with her against her husband and mother. Having run out of options, and looking for something else to try, one of them had made the referral.

The advantage of seeing triangles in this clinical situation is that it gave the therapist options that hadn't been tried before. First, the therapist assumed that, given Denise's history, there was a potentially significant triangle trap in this therapy, as there had been with Denise's other health care providers and her family. The therapist took some specific steps to avoid the triangle therapy trap in which Denise tried to get the therapist on her side against the husband–mother coalition. The therapist called the physician who was treating Denise's headaches and got his view of what was going on with the medical treatment and the psychological overlay. She reviewed with him how she saw the case and told him her plan to work with Denise's mother and husband. This greatly pleased the physician, who was tired of their constant interference and questioning of his treatment of Denise. Bringing Denise's mother and husband into sessions as "consultants" kept their potential reactivity to the therapist in check and calmed them down. Patients like Denise are too caught and powerless to be *coached* effectively on how to work their way out of these kinds of triangles. There is just not enough emotional resilience left after the relationship pressure and the depression have taken their toll. In clinical situations such as this, it is important to include the other two members of the triangle and to engage them in changing their part in the triangle's workings. This also reinforces the therapist's efforts to avoid becoming overly aligned with the patient, and preserves a critical level of objectivity.

The therapist worked to modify the triangle consisting of Denise, her husband, and her mother in sessions with each member. The anxiety that her mother and husband focused on Denise intensified her stress and decreased the effectiveness of pharmacological interventions for her headaches. The therapist made the mother's and husband's focus on Denise explicit and highlighted the way that attention aggravated and maintained the symptoms. She got Denise to talk about her experience of their focus on her and how it affected her. The therapist pointed out that with nothing but good intentions, Denise's husband and mother were giving her what they thought she needed: encouragement, advice, and instruction. The therapist suggested that this wasn't working, and recommended that they take time out to listen to Denise and allow her to tell them what she needs from them, and then try to provide it.

The therapist also asked Denise to listen to what her husband and mother needed from her. What they told her was that sometimes they thought she wasn't trying—that she wasn't compliant with her treatment and didn't really want to get better. When the therapist asked what gave them that impression, they replied that Denise didn't tell them anything. In fact, it was true that she often withdrew and shut down, probably in response to their instruction and criticism, and didn't tell them about what she was doing and how she was trying. Denise agreed to be more aggressive about communicating with them.

Eight weeks later, the therapist contacted Denise's physician to check on her progress. The physician reported that Denise hadn't had a headache for 2 weeks and that he was very encouraged. He also expressed his own relief that Denise's husband and mother were no longer on his back.

Connie—A Major Depression

Connie B. sought treatment for a symptom profile typical of a major depression. Over a 10-week period before calling for an appointment, she had noticed increasing levels of fatigue. She had spent long periods lying awake in bed, staring at the ceiling and thinking nothing but negative and morbid thoughts. When she began making excuses for not going to work, it had frightened her sufficiently that she decided to seek help. She went to her family physician, who had prescribed Prozac. She took it for 4 weeks with poor results. The family physician then referred her to a psychiatrist, who increased the dosage of medication and talked with her about the current stressors in her life. Suspecting marital problems, the psychiatrist referred her to a systems therapist.

In the evaluation session, Connie reported that this was the third such episode in her life. The first had occurred 16 years before when she was 16 and her next oldest sibling, Dale, had just left for college. That fall Connie had begun having academic difficulty in school, had lost interest in volleyball and dating, and had put on fifteen pounds. She remembered vividly the struggles with her mother over homework and the frustration her father experienced in the face of the constant bickering between them. Connie felt she had never measured up to what her mother wanted in a daughter. She always felt like an outsider in her relationships with her two older sisters, Joann, now 41, and Dale, now 34.

In fact, Connie never felt she fit in her family at all. As a youngster growing up in Westchester County, she was bigger than most of the young women her age, but she had superior athletic gifts. Besides volleyball, she had also excelled in lacrosse and swimming from an early age. This set her apart from her sisters, who were shorter and slimmer, specialized in looking pretty, and scored more than 1400 on their SAT's. Connie remembered longing to be better friends with her older sisters and wishing that her paternal grandmother were her mother. Grandma never criticized and always seemed to understand.

Connie's sisters had both graduated from Ivy League colleges and law schools and had settled in Washington, D.C. Both were married and had children and, to Connie, were living happily ever after. She found it ironic that her sisters had moved away and that she had settled in the same town in which she had grown up, since they had been such stars there, and she had been so unhappy. She never traveled very far, going to college at Sarah Lawrence in Westchester County, New York, and getting her master's in physical therapy in Manhattan. As an adolescent, mostly in the aftermath of conflicts with her mother, Connie would often fantasize about living in California. That fantasy ended, she guessed, when she met Justin at a New York City singles' bar while she was a graduate student. Justin was an older man, 30 when she met him; he owned his own business and was a "regular, quiet, but fun-loving guy." They courted for 2 years and after Connie finished her training, married and settled in Westchester. Justin's already thriving advertising and public relations business made California highly unlikely.

Two years after they married, Connie and Justin started thinking about having children, but when they stopped taking precautions, nothing happened. Halfway through a prolonged fertility work-up, Connie experienced her second episode of major depression. The hormonal rushes and emotional lability the fertility drugs produced in her were bad enough, but the lack of results was devastating. She remembered her grandmother, who had died when Connie was 13, telling her to take comfort in her size and strength because she would make healthy babies some day. She decided to stop trying to get pregnant for a while, and with the help of therapy and Prozac she felt somewhat better within 6 months.

During this time she recalls having noticed what was an increasing attachment between Justin and her mother. This pleased Connie greatly because it meant that her mother accepted Justin although he "wasn't Ivy League." Somehow in recent weeks, however, Connie had become increasingly annoyed at listening to Justin's encouragement and instructions each evening. It was very close to what felt like criticism from her mother.

Connie's life had been a series of sequential triangles. Born into the third and youngest sibling position in her family, she started out in the outside position in a triangle with her older sisters. Her sisters had been close, and they remained close all their lives—even settling in the same town, 250 miles from home, after law school. Being the outsider, as Connie was, is a vulnerable place to be for a kid who wants to be on the inside. In the triangle with her mother and sister she also occupied the outside position and was her mother's target child. The criticism from her mother was most intense during the period after Dale left for college. Somehow, Connie made it through, depressions and all.

Her present dilemma created the perfect mix for another bout of depression. If she took the fertility drugs, she'd have hormonal problems; if she didn't, she'd probably sacrifice reproductive function. As if that weren't enough, the activation of a triangle with her husband and mother completed the picture. As the systems therapist reviewed Connie's story, replete with all those triangles, it became clear that some sustained triangle work might improve Connie's response to Prozac, decrease the intensity of her intermittent bouts of depression, and give her the strength to try the fertility treatments again if she wants to.

THE THERAPY TRIANGLE

The therapy triangle occurs when a therapist becomes reactive to the emotional process either in the therapeutic relationship or in the family, and either takes sides or becomes paralyzed and unable to work effectively. Avoiding the therapy triangle when working with troubled marriages or with symptomatic children and their families is difficult enough. It is even more of a challenge in doing therapy with individuals. Having only one person in the room creates a level of empathy and identification that can ally the therapist inappropriately with the patient against the other people in the patient's life. Closing this chapter with some reflections on this problem seems appropriate.

Dealing with the therapy triangle means dealing with the relationship phenomena between patient, therapist, and significant others from the patient's life. In psychodynamic therapy, these phenomena are treated as transference and countertransference problems. It's relatively simple to shift one's viewpoint and see the phenomena of transference and countertransference as triangular phenomena. The advantage of doing so is that it gives the therapist increased options.

In the classical transference paradigm, the patient struggles with the universal problem of getting emotional needs met. In the process, they're confronted with conflicts between their internalized (intrapsychic) version of an important relationship object (for purposes of discussion, let's say it's their mother) and the reality object that's the mother they experience in everyday life. If the patient has a distorted internalized object—one in which she has overly idealized her mother—she may then expect her mother to deliver an abundance of nurturing supplies to her in the present. This leads to disappointment, hurt, and anger again and again. As the patient's dependency intensifies in the therapy relationship, the internalized version of mother gets externalized into the therapeutic relationship. The corresponding expectation of nurturing supplies from the therapist gets activated and once again is frustrated. The conflict between patient and mother is thereby transferred to the therapist. If we forget for a moment about the unconscious, we can see this phenomenon represents the displacement of needs and expectations from the mother to the therapist.

Displacement is one major mechanism of triangle activation. In systems psychotherapy, however, instead of encouraging the dependence of the patient on the therapist and thereby fostering the transference, we work to minimize the intensity of dependence within the therapeutic relationship and thereby try to minimize the transference. We achieve this by being active, real participants in the treatment relationship, by limiting the frequency of sessions, and by keeping the treatment focus on the patient's real-life relationships rather than on the relationship with the therapist. We also try to educate the patient about how a person's expectations are often not aligned with what the other person can realistically be expected to deliver. Finally, we send the patient back to work on the relationship with the significant other, or we bring the other into the therapy sessions.

It's not news that therapists are vulnerable to becoming emotionally reactive as they sort through a patient's situation and try to come up with a treatment plan that is effective and satisfactory to the patient. Most of us have spent time, energy, and money in our own therapy, in therapist's-own-family (TOF) work, or in supervision finding a way to handle our personal issues so that they don't compromise the treatment we provide. We've all been in situations in our clinical practice in which our own emotions, needs, biases, and assumptions blind us. Even in family and couple therapy, we get angry with one or more people in the treatment room for being difficult or resistant. We get caught in power struggles with some patients. Out of exasperation, we reactively and inappropriately label one patient as borderline and another narcissistic because we are unable to find a way around our lack of empathy. At other times, we're sometimes too empathetic with and protective of a patient. Our anxiety makes us overly responsible for patients' decisions and well-being. We work too hard and worry too much, unable to steer a clear path through our own reactivity, often paralyzing the patient in the process.

Usually when we look at these situations, we find countertransference issues. When we do, we can be confident that there are one or more therapy triangles we need to address. The therapist has a responsibility to search out countertransference reactions by actively attempting to understand them in the context of the therapist's own family. This is best done by getting supervision, clinical consultation, or coaching from a colleague, consultant, or therapist. However, many of the more minor countertransference reactions, if looked at as triangles, can be worked out by therapists themselves—locating their own triggers, calming their own reactivity, eliminating reactively driven behavior, and detriangling by putting the problem back into the context of the patient's life and helping the patient deal with it there.

One therapist requested a consultation for Eleanor, a 39-year-old divorced woman who had been seeing him in weekly psychotherapy for 10 months. Eleanor was talking in most sessions about her attraction to the therapist, her fantasies about him, and her lack of interest in meeting any other men. This woman had been utterly dependent on her husband, a thoroughly controlling man who had left her. The therapist had seen them both initially, and the husband left therapy almost immediately. The therapist was left with the devastated wife, who became increasingly dependent on the therapist and then eroticized the dependency. The therapist was anxious about the eroticized material, and his reactivity began because he didn't know what to do about it. He kept trying to convince the woman that she didn't feel this way, or that if she did, she shouldn't. The therapist's behavior was caused by his anxiety and his reactivity to the patient's displaced erotic feelings from her husband to him.

The consultant saw almost immediately that Eleanor's feelings for her therapist were a displacement of internal issues. She directly and without anxiety explored Eleanor's sexual fantasies about the therapist and with pointed questions linked them to unresolved issues concerning her husband. The consultant coached the therapist to stop running away from the patient and to start talking with her about it and what it meant in a way that made it safe for Eleanor to explore the feelings with the knowledge that at least one of them was in control. This advice was based on keeping the triangle in the consultant's consciousness: With ex-husband in the distant position, the wife was moving toward the therapist, and the therapist was distancing from the wife rather than standing still and dealing with her about her dependence on her husband. By seeing this as a triangular issue, and keeping the triangle in mind, the therapist was able to understand the emotional process, detoxify it, and encourage the patient to move on with her life and find new love objects, instead of focusing on a relationship in which her fantasies would never be realized.

The issue here isn't whether it's truth or fiction that we fall prey to in our role as healers, but rather, how we handle the emotional pressures that swirl around us in therapy and distort our vision. Here, the idea of the potential for a therapy triangle is invaluable in helping us keep our balance and therapeutic perspective. Moreover, understanding the manner in which you as a therapist can keep free of therapy triangles is critical to engaging the individuals you treat and to moving the therapy along. What is crucial is that by keeping out of triangles with your patients and their worlds, you become a person who is credible and safe for your patients.

The individual case studies in this chapter reveal the importance of understanding triangles in the formation of symptoms in the individual and the clinical management of these symptoms in the relationship context in which they occur. Having dealt with the individual, let's move on in the following chapters to deal with triangles involving married couples and children and adolescents in treatment.

CHAPTER NINE

Extrafamilial Triangles in Marital Conflict

Ann and David G. were both divorced and well into middle age when they met by chance through a mutual friend. Ann had promised herself that she would never remarry. She wanted to finish raising her children. David was only recently out of his marriage and busy adjusting to single parenthood. It was a surprise to both of them that after a few dates there was an intense bond forming between them. She loved his voice. He loved her smile. Two months later, they had declared their love. Six months after that, they were married, full of plans for the future, and excited about putting their families together. They felt sorry for others who didn't have what they had.

After a 3-day honeymoon in Vermont, Ann and David returned home to begin their new lives. Two weeks later, several hours before a party they were having for friends and family to celebrate their union, Ann was standing in the driveway crying and shrieking at David because his 7-year-old daughter had broken the bride and groom off the wedding cake. David ignored her. He was busy with Ann's ex-husband, who had arrived uninvited and drunk. The upset escalated, and David took his daughter by the hand as he stormed out of the house.

Ann and David made up after a miserable and anxious afternoon. They chalked up the fight to stress. However, over the next few months, the couple found themselves in increasing turmoil. David was feeling irritated with Ann, who left him notes as she went to work listing things she wanted him to do. He was annoyed while he prepared meals the kids wouldn't eat and drove them to their activities. He dreaded answering the phone because Ann's ex-husband or ex-mother-in-law often called at night when Ann was working. Even the family dog seemed to demand David's attention.

Meanwhile, Ann worked often at night, when her family responsibilities were the greatest. She was relieved that her new husband could take up the slack for her and was particularly happy that her children now had a functioning father. Her only disappointment was that David seemed uninterested in making love. Before they married, he couldn't keep his hands off her.

One night Ann had it out with David. Tearfully she described her upset that he had not touched her in weeks. David shot back that he was sick and tired of her bossiness. Ann was shocked. David refused to talk to her and rolled over and was snoring before she had taken her pillows and blanket to the couch in the den.

How is it that this couple, who were so in love and full of excitement, got into such a state and so soon in their marriage? They had started as a close and loving twosome, but it became evident early on that their twosome wasn't really a twosome at all: It was really many threesomes, constantly changing the two of them. One answer to this question is that marital conflict involves triangles. Always. Sometimes, these are very intense; usually there are several operating at once.

You're familiar with the extramarital affair triangle, the mother-in-law triangle, and the child triangle born with the first child. Less familiar and less obvious are those other triangles that also bind the subtle and not-so-subtle conflicts between husband and wife. Triangles organize marital conflict, providing a focus for it, and often they cover up emotional problems in the marriage itself. Examples are the woman who adores her father and is never satisfied with her husband's accomplishments or the wife who isn't interested in sex when her child leaves for college or her mother's cancer goes out of remission.

Marital triangles are formed when the partners don't resolve the differences between them. The implicit or explicit relationship debris, when ignored, makes fertile soil for triangulation either within the family or externalized and projected outside the family. There are seven main types of triangles in marital conflict, most of which have variations or subtypes. Of the seven main types, three, extramarital affairs, social network triangles, and occupational triangles, are extrafamilial. Four are intrafamilial: in-law triangles, triangles with the children, spouse and sibling triangles, and the primary parental triangle of each spouse. Extrafamilial triangles are usually activated because the system cannot deal with one or more intrafamilial triangles.

Extrafamilial triangles usually represent the externalization of a dysfunctional process going on within the family. When the clinician sees extrafamilial triangles, she or he can assume two things. First, they're connected to an intrafamilial triangle or to an interlocking set of intrafamilial triangles. Second, the multigenerational family unit has been unable to contain the reactive emotional process in that triangle or set of triangles. The result is that the process spills out and incorporates people from outside the system by forming an extrafamilial triangle.

THE EXTRAMARITAL AFFAIR TRIANGLE

There are as many reasons why people end up in affairs as there are affairs. People are frequently surprised to find themselves in such a spot. "It was just one of those things, just one of those crazy things," says the song. Whatever the trigger—midlife crisis, a need to be understood, a desire for an exotic sexual escapade, tension release, a transition out of a marriage—most people don't plan their affairs, at least not consciously. Often the most uncomfortable partner is the one to begin the affair—including the retaliatory affair—the payback for the affair the other person has had.

An affair is not a symptom of a character disorder. People rarely intend to cause the other person pain, even if anger, hurt, or loneliness is the fuel for the breaking of the trust. An extramarital affair is an effort to reduce discomfort and anxiety by externalizing into an affair the unresolved problems between two people. Two examples are the excluded husband in a triangle with his wife and children, and the wife who receives constant criticism from both her husband and her mother.

An affair can have several effects on a marriage. One possibility is that the affair can calm down the uncomfortable partner without disturbing the other spouse, thus stabilizing the marriage and covering over its underlying dysfunction. This effect is often temporary and usually ends when the other spouse finds out about the affair.

A second possibility is that upon discovery the affair itself becomes the central issue between the spouses. Then the affair covers over the conflictual process in the marriage that triggered the affair in the first place. When the affair is an open issue, it is especially important for the therapist to remember the distinction between being part of a relationship process and being responsible for one's own behavior. In the extramarital affair triangle, the participating spouse must take responsibility for his or her behavior and not attempt to excuse it because of preexisting relationship problems. On the other hand, both spouses must take responsibility for their parts in the relationship process that preceded the affair.

A third possibility is that the covering-over function of the affair isn't totally successful. Here, the couple present for treatment around other issues with the affair still a secret. This situation raises the thorny issue of confidentiality for the therapist.

If the therapist learns of the affair, she or he must decide whether to raise the affair in a conjoint session. While some writers[1] make a theoretical argument about the desirability of total openness for revealing the affair, it is our position that this should not generally be done. Informing the ignorant spouse of the affair will raise the couple's anxiety at the very point in treatment when a major goal is to reduce anxiety. The major exception to this rule is the case in which the ignorant spouse, convinced that something is going on but confronted with constant denial, is becoming severely depressed or even psychotic.

Therapists' Tasks in Affair Triangles

Few topics generate the kind of strong feelings and inflamed discussion among therapists as extramarital affairs. Therapists who are in affairs themselves, or feel victimized by someone who has had an affair (a partner, a parent), may take extreme positions for or against the acceptability of such behavior. As with most emotional issues, therapists need to be clear about their own biases in order to be most helpful to the couples they see. If they can't, they will surely create intense therapy triangles by siding with the offended spouse or secretly applauding the offender. When therapists learn of an affair, they face three important tasks. The first is to make a clinical judgment about whether to make a "secret" affair, past or present, clinically explicit. The second is to make it clear to the spouse having the affair that he or she must end the affair if the couple is to make progress in marital therapy. Third, while doing this, the therapist must also recognize

---

[1]For example, Pittman (1989).

and validate the pain and sense of loss that the person having an affair will experience. This is done in sessions alone with the participating spouse.

The extramarital affair triangle raises some of the most interesting and challenging issues that a therapist who works with marital conflict encounters. One of the authors faced the following clinical situations within a 1-year period. A married woman came for therapy alone to address the fact that she had been having an affair for 7 years, a fact that remained unknown to her husband. She died during emergency surgery after several months of therapy, and following her death, her distraught husband sought treatment to deal with the loss. His idealization of his wife and of the marriage was interfering with the grieving process and his return to good functioning. In another case, the therapist knew that an 8-year-old daughter was the offspring of the wife's lover rather than of her husband. In a third case, the therapist was working with two couples who were friends. He learned that the wife of one was having an affair with the husband of the other.

Although these cases were particularly dramatic, we focus our approach to treatment in each case with an extramarital affair triangle on the following goals:

1. *Alter the emotional climate between the couple by calming them down.* Do this by normalizing the issues and give them tasks aimed at treating each other with decency while working on the problem in therapy.

2. *Change each person's behavior around the affair.* For example, the spouse who is having an ongoing affair needs to end it. The therapist may have to take time allowing this person to grieve the loss in sessions without his or her partner. The spouse who has not had the affair may be checking up all the time on his wife, or demanding to have the details of the sexual relationship between the lovers. This behavior needs to stop.

3. *Systematize the affair.* Each partner has played a part in making the marriage fertile ground for an affair to develop. This isn't to say that the betrayed spouse is as guilty as the spouse who has cheated. It is a way of equalizing responsibility for the emotional state of the marriage—which helped fuel the anxiety out of which come triangles like affairs. By systematizing the affair, the therapist can address the unresolved conflict and distance that are at the root of the triangle.

4. *Work on the intrafamilial triangles that appear.* As the work progresses on dismantling the affair triangle, intrafamilial triangles will become more apparent. These triangles, operating within the ex-

tended or nuclear family, usually predate the affair but have not been exposed or resolved. They add to the fuel in the affair triangle.

5. *Reestablish trust and credibility.* Do this by dealing with the betrayed partner's anxieties and need to ask questions. The one who had the affair has to take responsibility for his or her actions and express remorse for them. Therapy should also explore the symmetrical trust issue (see below).

The couples who do best with the extramarital affair triangle have four key characteristics. They come to understand the process that led up to the affair and the part that each played in it. They shift their respective positions in the current process. They move slowly and thoughtfully toward a new kind of trust and intimacy in the marital relationship. Finally, they come to understand their scripting from their families of origin. Here's an example.

Ed and Linda G. met and dated in college. Linda got pregnant in her junior year and had an abortion. They married in 1984, 3 years after Ed's graduation. They now had one child, Laurie, who was 3 years old at the time the couple came to therapy. Linda had just found out about Ed's 9-month affair with Nadine—an affair that had ended when Nadine aborted a pregnancy.

Ed was a 32-year-old marketing manager for a local subsidiary of a large corporation. For some time, he had been living with the constant fear that the corporate headquarters located 1,000 miles away would sell or close the subsidiary, and he would lose his job. He was the oldest of four children, and the only son. He loved sports and was himself a talented athlete who placed great importance on playing golf and league baseball very well. Both of Ed's parents were living and were 60 years old. His mother was in good health and worked as a secretary. His father had been retired on disability for 8 years; he had a serious neuromuscular disease that made him an invalid much of the time. Tears welled up in Ed's eyes when he told the therapist that his father didn't have much time left and could die at any time. Ed idealized his parents and was reluctant to say anything negative about them, but Linda interrupted to say that Ed's parents had always made him believe that "he's a piece of shit."

Linda was the youngest of four sisters and a twin. She worked as a human resources manager for a midsize manufacturing company. Her father, with whom she had been close, had died when she was in college of the same disease Ed's father was now suffering from. Her mother had remarried, and no one in the family (except, presumably,

Linda's mother) liked her current husband. Linda said that her mother had had an affair during her father's years of illness.

The therapist asked about Ed's affair. Ed told him that Nadine was the wife in a couple who had been friends of his and Linda's since shortly after they were married. They were also neighbors and regularly saw quite a bit of each other. Ed said that an "attraction" between him and Nadine had begun the previous Thanksgiving, and at the time of the neighborhood Christmas party, they had snuck off to begin their sexual liaison. Privately, Ed described the sex as intensely gratifying. Obviously, Ed's theory about the reasons for, or the origin of, the affair centered on his wife's unwillingness to have sex as often as he wanted. Linda's view of the affair was complex. She blamed Ed's parents in part, because they had always torn Ed down, and he needed constant building up. "I got tired of doing that, and Nadine did it," she said. She also blamed herself, agreeing with Ed that her "low sex drive" since Laurie's birth had created a real problem in the marriage. When the therapist asked about the status of Ed's relationship with Nadine, both told him it was over. He had had no contact with Nadine at all since her abortion, and he expressed great fear about seeing her. He said he believed that Nadine was responsible for some hangup telephone calls he had received at work, and the thought that she might be trying to reach him upset him greatly. He was afraid that she'd say things that would make him feel like a heel.

The fact that the affair was over solved one problem confronting the clinician in the early stages of an affair case: *taking a position that the affair must end.* Evidently this one already had. If it hadn't, the therapist would have explained that marital therapy was a waste of time and money while the affair continued. The therapist would then have monitored Ed's emotional state, knowing that, if he were following the contract, he would be sad or angry.

Another problem of the early stage of treatment in these cases is encouraging the betrayed spouse to figure out what behavior she or he won't tolerate and what she or he can't live with. Then the betrayed spouse must *pull back to a nonreactive position.* Linda let Ed know that any repetition of his infidelity would mean the end of the marriage. Fidelity was her one nonnegotiable demand. Her ability to pull back to a nonreactive position, to refrain from pursuing Ed with questions and recriminations, wasn't so easy. However, she saw very clearly the importance to their recovery of doing so, and she went to work on this task with energy and determination. Her success or failure had to be monitored every week in therapy; in Linda's case, her "slips" took the form of occasional questions and "looking depressed."

In another task essential to the early stages of therapy, the therapist had to help Ed *grieve the loss.* Ed denied he felt any loss, except perhaps the loss of Nadine's admiration and praise. However, he was putting significant pressure on Linda for immediate forgiveness *and* for plenty of sex. Linda complained about that, and the therapist worked at getting Ed to pull back from his pressuring without getting angry or emotionally distant. Ed agreed to work on this, but it was a real struggle, and when he was successful at it he got mildly depressed.

Given Ed and Linda's commitment to each other, and the fact that the affair was unequivocally over, these steps quickly stabilized their emotional state and calmed the marital climate. Ed continued to have bouts of discouragement and depression stemming largely from self-pity when he was successful at not pressuring Linda. Linda continued to feel hurt and angry when she thought of the affair and resentful when Ed pressured her for forgiveness and sex. Nevertheless, the couple's behavior with one another was calmer.

As the therapist explored their continuing efforts to deal with the affair's fallout, he discovered several patterns that Ed and Linda agreed had long been problems for them. Ed admitted that he engaged in a pattern of fear, anger, and withdrawal. Ed would be afraid of not being perfect, of failure, of feeling bad. Then he would blame Linda for her lack of encouragement, support, and sex. Finally, he would withdraw into silence and lack of effort and responsibility for the relationship. Linda admitted that what she perceived as Ed's neediness frightened her. She said that she would prefer to withdraw in the face of a problem or demand and let it fester.

The therapist helped Linda and Ed trace these patterns back to their primary parental triangles and to the roles each of them had played in those triangles. Ed had been the "target child"[2]—the object of parental criticism and concern—and had always felt undervalued and unsupported. Linda had been her father's special child, an emotional substitute for a wife who couldn't deal with her husband's illness and weakness.

The therapist also helped them devise methods for shifting these patterns. They included Ed paying attention to Linda at dinnertime so that she could talk to him about her day, her worries, her news.

---

[2]See Guerin and Gordon (1984).

The therapist helped Ed to realize that his sexual demands only made Linda more distant and negative toward him. Ed agreed to concentrate on being affectionate and interested in Linda in a nonsexual context. Linda had often expressed in sessions how little energy Ed put into their relationship unless he wanted sex. She was suspicious when he was "nice" and wanted him to be interested in all of her.

Linda was to give Ed a few minutes alone when she came home (he got out of work first and took responsibility for Laurie's care and entertainment). She was also to take responsibility for their sex life—to initiate sex (something she rarely did) when she was feeling sexual. These plans worked fairly well. Among other things, Linda got in touch with her sex drive, which was not as "low" as she had thought (or as high as Ed hoped it would be). Sex continued to be difficult for them but with a lower level of hurt and resentment on both sides. Now they could listen without reactivity to each one's vulnerability and point of view about sex.

A second process leading up to the affair centered on the triangle with their daughter, Laurie. Both Ed and Linda agreed that their problems really began after Laurie's birth when Linda experienced a lowering of her interest in sex. She also felt considerable guilt, or at least uncertainty, about her decision to return to work immediately. Ed's fear of failure and need to be perfect intensified now that he was a father. He wanted to be the perfect father. Further, Ed and Linda disagreed about how they should raise Laurie. When Laurie had a tantrum, for example, Ed lost his patience and yelled at her; Linda stepped in to defend her. Ed spoke of the need to "train" Laurie not to be bad (as he had been), while Linda read child-care books and said things such as, "It's normal." "It's just a phase." "She'll get over it."

Again these behaviors were traced back to Ed's and Linda's families Ed said that, deep down, he believed that he would never have straightened out if his parents hadn't been strict with him. As much as he resented the damage their criticism had done to him, he found himself doing what they had done. Linda saw that, like her mother, she preferred not to vocalize problems and to act as if everything were okay, ignoring any opinions to the contrary. Linda was particularly leery of any interpretation (by herself or by Ed) of Laurie's behavior that might suggest that her job (which she loved) was interfering with her mothering.

Understanding more about their families motivated Ed and Linda to moderate their behavior toward Laurie. In addition, they worked out with the therapist some structural detriangling moves that the therapist hoped would reinforce the new team approach. First, the therapist pointed out to Ed that he had idealized his father and that this contributed to his treating Laurie as his father had treated him. Just as he had never satisfied his father with anything he did—grades, sports, or the woman he married—Ed was on the same critical path with his daughter. First, the therapist suggested that Ed get a more personal (and therefore more balanced) relationship with his father. Ed was to go to his father and talk to him about his (Ed's) negativity and pessimism. In addition, the therapist instructed each of them to stay out of the other's relationship with Laurie. Since abuse of any kind was not even in question here, the therapist pointed out that each of them had to have his or her own relationship with Laurie, and had to take personal responsibility for how that relationship turned out.

Ed and Linda each took responsibility for their part of the problem with Laurie. Ed addressed his reactivity with his father, Laurie, and Linda. Linda began to look at her guilt for having a career and her tendency to bury her head in the sand like her mother. Instead of blaming Ed, she began to acknowledge that she had a good deal of ambivalence about balancing her needs with those of her child. Meanwhile, tension from the affair waxed and waned depending on the stress in the system. The tension increased, for example, whenever they thought that Nadine was calling and hanging up, or asking mutual friends about them. It increased 8 months into therapy, when Ed's father died. It also increased around the anniversary of Linda's discovery of the affair. When this happens, it is important to reassure the couple by normalizing such fluctuations and to coach them to use the tools they now have to deal with this fallout.

Rebuilding Credibility

The therapist asked Linda what she needed to start trusting Ed again. She said that it was difficult for her when he went out; she would experience doubts about where he was and whom he was with. Linda said that if Ed told her where he was going, who would be there, and what time he would be home, that would help. Ed said that doing that would be like having a jailer: It would remind him of reporting to his mother as an adolescent. Nevertheless, he said that he saw how important it could be and that he would gladly do it. He did so, faithfully. Then he got angry when Linda continued to have doubts and worries when he went out. The therapist pointed out to Ed that he couldn't expect to rebuild credibility with Linda all at once; he had to build a record of trustworthiness, and that takes time. Ed reluctantly agreed.

Asking for Details

This is a thorny problem. When couples first come to therapy, we typically find the betrayed spouse pursuing the other one with detailed questions about the affair and the third party. Simultaneously, the spouse who had the affair is resentful of the questions and gets defensive and distant. Timing is everything. Answering Linda's questions too early in the healing process would surely cause major upset for her. On the other hand, answering questions can be helpful when enough repair has taken place that it would help Linda to have a more realistic picture of the relationship between Nadine and Ed. In the controlled milieu of the therapy room, the therapist can give the betrayed spouse the chance to ask his or her questions without using them to attack and berate the other spouse. The other spouse ought to answer them. If he or she is unwilling to answer, the reestablishment of trust is set back, because it appears that the guilty spouse is protecting the third party.

When Ed and Linda and the therapist came to this point in therapy, Linda said she had no questions. She didn't want to ask anything, wasn't curious about any of the details. Ed said that, painful as it might be to "rehash things," he was willing to answer any questions she had. The therapist told Linda that having questions was normal, and explained that, at this stage of treatment, dealing with them might be productive. Linda remained adamant, however, that she had no questions at this time. The therapist chose to accept her reluctance, fitting in as it did with her avoidant style. He checked in with Linda in future sessions to encourage her to ask. In an individual session with her the therapist probed her lack of curiosity. She said that she had made peace with not knowing, that it was more comfortable for her.

Taking Responsibility and Expressing Remorse

If a person who has an affair blames someone else or claims that she or he did nothing wrong, forget reestablishing trust. This wasn't Ed's position. From the beginning he blamed himself and expressed deep remorse. Far from denying responsibility, Ed overreacted: his remorse became self-hatred, verging on self-pity. The problem when the person who had the affair takes a too negative view of self because of the affair is that *it serves to perpetuate the affair triangle although the affair itself is over.* Having a "saint and sinner" mentality continues the triangle, although the third point is now the affair itself rather than the lover. The affair becomes the deed around which the husband and wife now dance. This makes total sense, of course, if we see the function of triangles as stabilization of an unstable dyad.[3] A *realistic* view and acknowledgment of one's responsibility, and the expression of *appropriate* remorse is necessary to put the affair triangle behind the couple. Ed found that difficult to do. Altering the triangular structure is impossible unless both partners can see their own and the other's contribution to the unresolved conflict in the marriage.

Frequently the betrayed spouse perpetuates the triangle by placing all or most of the blame on the third party. Rather than holding the spouse responsible for the infidelity, the betrayed spouse lays the blame at the feet of the lover. This is another version of taking all the blame for oneself. It's skewed and unrealistic, and even disrespectful. Is the betrayer so inept and helpless that the lover captured him or her? Linda tended to absolve Ed and give Nadine more responsibility for the affair. She expressed "hatred" of Nadine. "How could a woman do a thing like that? How could she have an affair with a friend's husband?" This of course had the unintended consequence of keeping Nadine in their lives mentally and emotionally, though she was gone physically. The best way to get her out, of course, is to see her as a *person,* with assets and limitations, and with a life history, just like everyone else. People can rarely hear this from a therapist, and so people rarely fully disentangle themselves from an affair triangle.

The Symmetrical Trust Issue

The unfaithful spouse invariably has an underground trust issue with the betrayed spouse. In Ed's case, the symmetrical trust issue centered on sex. Ed found it difficult to trust that Linda really cared about their sex life and his sexual needs, and that she would really try to make it better, because for years she had avoided him in the bedroom. It was when they began to work on this that Ed and Linda, at Linda's urging, decided to end therapy. It was 13 months from the time they first came.

---

[3]Fogarty (1975).

SOCIAL NETWORK TRIANGLES

These triangles involve people outside the family system as the third parties. A common complaint from people is that their spouses are involved with friends who are "giving them the wrong ideas." Triangles are often a matter of influence, and this is especially true with a social network triangle. We may describe a triangle as a competition of influences. If you doubt the power of this dynamic, just remember the last time you brought home some opinion only to hear your partner remind you, all hurt, that he or she had been telling you that for years! We strive for autonomy, but often, we end up migrating back and forth among different sources of connection and influence.

No one—except the two people involved—believes that marriage makes partners put the opinions of their spouses ahead of the opinions of everyone else. Couples expect it of each other, however unreasonable that expectation appears to an outside observer. For example, a wife begins at some point to turn her attention to personal self-fulfillment. Along the way, she may form a relationship with a woman whose beliefs may conflict with those of her husband. As this friend raises her consciousness, a potent triangle is activated. If the husband is conservative in his outlook, the conflict will be overt and the battle for dominance of influence will be right on the surface.

On the other hand, if the husband is of a more liberal persuasion, the conflict will be more subtle. The husband who is supportive of his wife's career, equality, and independence, becomes reactive to the loss he feels when part of his wife's attention and emotional investment is directed elsewhere. When, as often happens, the husband is an emotional distancer, his wife's not being where he would like her to be creates internal discomfort. Because it is not intellectually acceptable to be upset at his wife's movement or to be angry at the new influence on her, the conflict is often expressed in covert ways. He is an intellectual egalitarian and an emotional traditionalist.

Her expectations that her liberal husband and informed children will applaud her movement toward self-actualization often trip up the wife in this situation. They do of course, but within limits, and these limits are defined by their own levels of internal discomfort and their need for her to take care of them.

Therapists must be alert to how their own emotional triggers may set up a therapy triangle in response to a position one spouse is taking with another about outside influence. For example, a therapist sought supervision for a case with a very controlling, fiscally tight husband and a compliant, nonassertive, and financially underresponsible wife. The therapist, who happened to be a woman, found herself pushing the husband to disclose their assets to his wife. One could say that the therapist was only trying to create openness and balance in the couple's power struggle about money. That might have been true. Nevertheless, the therapist was aware on some level that she was annoyed with the husband's behavior, and it reminded her of a triangle she had been (and still was) in with her own extended family. Her father spent money flamboyantly, while her mother hoarded and saved every cent she could, especially the money she took from her husband's wallet when he was sleeping.

Another instance was the therapist who felt almost fatherly toward one wife as he encouraged her to get a graduate degree and ignored or labeled as invalid her husband's complaints that his wife was never available to him or their children. The therapist here was playing out the triangle in his marriage to a wife he didn't respect because she never did anything "intellectual" and her closest two friends had never been to college.

Understanding the triangles in your own family is critical to being able to work adequately with relationship triangles in therapy. How do you know you're caught? When you are having a strong emotional response to either partner, when you don't know what questions to ask, or when you begin to take sides. Naturally, we're people with relationships before we're therapists. We need to remember that we're just as vulnerable to ending up in triangles with patients as they are with other people in their lives. We must be in touch with our emotional reactivity even when we are intellectually committed to equality between the sexes.

As marriages continue to evolve from the traditional model to a more egalitarian style, many younger couples are struggling to find a way of being equal partners and developing an understanding of how each partner can remain an individual even as they work to become a couple. How explicit their understandings are depends largely on the couple's political philosophies, the characteristics of their social networks, and where in the country they live. The question of influence is important in all marriages, however, and the therapist must be diligent in looking for influence triangles when dealing with marital conflict.

The bond between marital partners has an expectation of loyalty that is present in no other relationship. When one spouse believes that bond has been broken, and that an outsider is in the position the spouse should be in, the resulting jealousy and resentment are profound. Take Don and Sue, for example. Don had been sober in AA for several years, and he and his wife were in therapy because they were fighting over many issues. One issue in particular concerned Sue's Al-Anon group, who, Don believed, were poisoning Sue's attitude toward him. He accused them of being "a bunch of dried-up old bitches," who were telling her not to have sex with him and coaching her to be selfish and ungenerous. Sue's response to this was to attack Don and his AA buddies, who often got together for coffee after their meetings. To her, they were male chauvinists. Don and Sue's attachment to their respective groups, and the intense triangles they were in, kept them from dealing with the issues of change in their relationship now that Don's drinking had stopped. The fighting also provided a place for them to act out their anger and hurt, with which they had never dealt.

Another form the social network triangle can take is a triangle with friends who predate the marriage. A husband stays connected with his college roommates after the marriage. They meet twice a year in New York to spend the weekend drinking and going to strip joints. His wife may see these activities and their importance as infringing on the time her husband has for her and the children. She resents her husband's adolescent behavior under the influence of these friends and suspects that there might be sexual high jinks on these outings. The prescribed clinical protocol is to help couples like this sort out the problems of influence, individual versus couple and family time, and the underlying difficulty, always present, of balancing closeness and distance.

Other competing influences that can activate the social network triangle include such things as sports activities, clubs, community activities, or a mentor–disciple relationship. Spotting the triangle is usually quite simple because the reactive spouse is usually vocal about his or her belief that the third person or group takes up far too much of the spouse's time and is probably brainwashing the spouse in some way.

Dorothy S. was married to Ron, an attorney who went to law school early in their marriage and was supported by Dorothy. Dorothy didn't mind the work. She was a nurse in a large hospital in New York, and she believed that when Ron finished school and set up his practice they would finally have time together. After he graduated and passed the bar Ron spent many hours away from home getting his practice off the ground. Dorothy told herself that this was temporary and poured herself into raising their four children. Ron's practice became very successful, and he decided to use his leisure time to take up long-distance running. He was a good athlete and had run track in college. Before long he joined a local track club and began training for the New York Marathon. Ron spent many hours a week running with his club mates, and every Sunday he would enter a local race with his club. He urged Dorothy to attend his races, and sometimes she did, but she was becoming angry and resentful, tired of always waiting for him. She liked golf and had hoped he would play with her now that they could afford a country club membership.

At night Ron would end up falling asleep in front of the television exhausted from his workouts. The kids thought their Dad was "cool"; Dorothy thought he was cold, obsessed, and selfish. To make matters worse, running was all Ron ever talked about. Ron also decided to become a vegetarian, and his already lean frame became leaner. Dorothy, who had a tendency to gain weight anyway, gained 43 pounds. Ron made no bones about how much he disliked fat women. Dorothy and Ron fought constantly about Ron's involvement with running and the club and about Dorothy's weight. They dreaded weekends.

It is common to have one spouse blame the marital unhappiness or spouse's neglect on the latest fad or activity, or on the people with whom the spouse engages in that activity. The blaming is particularly intense when the people involved have a long history with the spouse, even predating the marriage.

One of the authors remembers a case that occurred early in her career that brought home this lesson. A young and newly married couple came for marital therapy. They had been married only 5 months when they got into a ferocious battle over the husband's softball practice and games. The husband reported that they had met in a bar after one of his games, which she had attended. During their courtship the couple had spent a great deal of their dating time involved with his softball league. She never missed a game, nor did she complain about his many practices and the traditional trip to the bar afterwards.

One night after they were married, during spring training, the wife demanded of her husband an explanation of where he was going. He was walking through the kitchen in his uniform as she was cooking dinner. "I'm going to softball practice, of course." "Oh no you're not," she retorted. He accused her of changing the rules on him when she said, "You're my husband now, and the marriage comes first." He was angry and confused, and they engaged daily in a power struggle over his softball commitment. The husband's friends had gone from being a part of their lives to the "enemy" in a few short months. Dealing with this triangle was necessary before the therapist could get access to the emotional process fueling the power struggle between these two newlyweds.

Sally P. had been an avid amateur apiarist since her early 20s, long before she met and married Gene. They had been married for 2 years, and Gene had always been fascinated by her hobby and impressed with her knowledge. They had even planned their honeymoon to coincide with an international conference for beekeepers in Spain. Later Gene was stunned (not stung) when he found Sally more interested in bees than in him. She spent many hours a week talking with other apiarists and went on excursions to see other hives in the area. Gene has found himself so frustrated with Sally that he has had fantasies of setting fire to her hives. He now refused to eat the honey from the hives, although he had once enjoyed it on his morning toast. Now, it made him ill.

In this triangle as in others, encouraging Gene to neutralize his reactivity and to begin to understand how the triangle operated and the function it served in the marriage are the first step in detriangling it and finding the problem between Gene and Sally. In this situation, Gene and Sally had married for the first time in their 40s. Both had been loners and enjoyed their space. The issue of the beekeeping and all it brought with it was deflecting the couple's attention from the difficulty they were having in becoming a couple. Their discomfort with being together and their difficulty negotiating their differences and their space were underlying the beekeeping issue. Neither could see or talk about his or her discomfort with being married. The therapist made it safe for them to discuss their expectations and disappointments. She normalized their feelings and validated their concerns. She helped them place the third point in the triangle (beekeeping and other beekeepers) in perspective and coached them to talk directly and constructively with one another.

The therapist also teased out the relevant issues in their families of origin that had contributed to the way Gene and Sally related to each other. Both had grown up in families where their parents never talked about anything that might be the least bit upsetting. Gene's father was a violent alcoholic, and his mother had tried to keep things calm. Sally's mother had been an invalid. She had had multiple sclerosis for many years, and Sally as the oldest daughter took care of her father and her three sisters. She came to love her privacy, and she "knew" that one should not make waves lest she upset someone she loved. Gene and Sally were extremely responsible but burdened people.

As Sally and Gene slowly learned to talk about the families in which they grew up, listening to each other and learning about one another, they began to notice and comment that they really were "made for each other." They had both been in the same position in their families of origin, and both believed that no news was the best news. Both began to understand that the position they occupied between their parents and among their brothers and sisters was a way to keep themselves calm when things got chaotic. They also saw, however, that that position contributed to isolation, distance, and loneliness. Learning to let go of their need to be in that place let them become a couple.

OCCUPATIONAL TRIANGLES

Complaints about a partner's preoccupation with work are extremely common. One way of looking at these grievances is to see if the job itself is the third leg of the triangle or if the work triangle involves a third person, whose attachment the other spouse resents. What's important to remember in these cases is that it's the emotional process that counts. A very close relationship with someone other than the marital partner, even if it isn't sexual, can be as intense a triangle as an affair.

Mark and Jessica Z. came to therapy with Jessica seething over Mark's unwillingness to set some limits with Lewis, his boss. Lewis called the house at least once a day. Often these calls came just as Mark pulled into the driveway. The children, who were 5 and 6, would be jumping up and down wanting to see Dad, who was on the phone with Lewis sometimes for over an hour. Lately Jessica had become so angry over Mark's refusal to take her upset seriously that she couldn't even be civil to Lewis when he called. Twice, she confessed, she had told Lewis that Mark wasn't home when she heard him drive into the garage.

Mark couldn't believe how Jessica was behaving. Lewis had given them money for the mortgage on their house, had bankrolled their business, and took Mark on fabulous ski trips because Lewis didn't like to travel alone. Mark pointed out that Jessica didn't mind spending the money or enjoying the prosperous life style that his relationship with Lewis provided. Jessica wanted a divorce. She couldn't tolerate Mark's attitude about her complaints or his loyalty to Lewis.

Jessica and Mark went on to an acrimonious divorce. Neither could get the overheated emotionality under control enough to begin to see the automatic dance that went on over Lewis. Mark couldn't empathize with Jessica, whom he saw as jealous and spiteful, virtually biting the hand that fed her. Jessica, however, continued to be outraged. Mark had no qualms about moaning and groaning when Lewis treated him badly. She thought she was about number 10 on Mark's list of priorities. So, she demanded that they sell their house and buy another one without any involvement from Lewis or his money. Mark refused, and the dance continued until they became irrevocably distant.

If therapy had succeeded in altering the emotional climate between Mark and Jessica, and in engaging their minds and efforts to change the movement in the triangle with Lewis, the therapist would have had the chance to coach them to behave differently. For example, Jessica might have tried moving toward Lewis rather than away: engaging him in conversation, inviting him to dinner (just as you might if your son or daughter is dating someone you don't like), asking Mark Lewis-oriented questions and saying things like "What does Lewis think about this?" or "How would Lewis solve that problem?" That would have been a way for Jessica consciously to alter her part in the triangle and free herself from the sort of automatic emotional response that fuels the feelings of helplessness and victimization.

The spouse who travels a good deal of the time isn't around when the partner or family needs him or her. Spouses who experience this kind of work-related loneliness often say they feel like single parents. The employee who talks about a colleague at work *ad nauseam,* disciples who work closely with mentors they sometimes think of as godlike, the difficult job situation whose demands the employed spouse is finding it difficult to meet and so has it running his family life are all examples of occupational triangles. In American society, where work is prized and success is important, we don't see it as valid to criticize a spouse's overinvolvement with the work system. Work then breeds resentment and labels the complaining spouse inappropriately jealous. It's not as if the spouse involved with work is being unfaithful, but the partners on the outside of this triangle often experience the occupational involvement as a breach of loyalty to them and to the family. It is the therapist's job to unearth the emotional process underlying this triangle and provide some balance and reality for both people.

When a marital case comes to therapy with an extrafamilial triangle in the foreground, its resolution is sometimes all the couple needs to be ready to work directly on their relationship. Usually, however, resolving extrafamiliar triangles uncovers the intrafamiliar triangles with which they are connected and which they allow a couple to avoid. We turn now to a consideration of intrafamilial marital triangles.

CHAPTER TEN

Marital Triangles within the Family

We have divided the most common triangles of marital conflict that occur within families into family-of-origin triangles and nuclear family triangles. The former include in-law triangles, spouse and sibling triangles, and the primary parental triangle of each spouse. Nuclear family triangles are those that involve one or more of the children.

Family-of-origin triangles are those involving one or both spouses and a member or members of their own families. The extended family triangles that predominate clinically are the in-law triangles, spouse and sibling triangles, and the primary parental triangle of each spouse. The extended family triangles that surround a marriage are by-products of three factors: primacy of attachment, hierarchy of influence, and displacement of conflict.

PRIMACY OF ATTACHMENT
AND HIERARCHY OF INFLUENCE

The formation of the marital bond requires spouses to shift their primary emotional attachment from the relationship with their parents to the relationship with their mates. If this shift takes place in a functional way, the relationship with parents remains intact. Over time, it's replaced in its primacy by the relationship with one's marital partner. A variety of problems develop as couples attempt to accomplish this shift. The form these problems take greatly influences the structure of extended family triangles.

As the attempt to shift the primary attachment is taking place in the courtship and early part of the marriage, a battle often follows over hierarchy of influence. Loyalty to one's clan becomes an issue. Which family's value system and way of doing things will prevail is a question not only for the partners but also for their families. An undergraduate student of one of the authors wrote the following in an assignment:

> My father always reminds my brother and my sister and me that "No matter what, always stay close with each other because your spouses may try to bring us apart from one another." He and my mother say to us, "Your immediate family comes first because those are your roots. Your wives or your husbands may try to tell you how wrong your brother or your sister or your mother is, but don't let them tear you apart from your family because that's all you have." I think that what my dad says is right. I love my family very much and I can see my brothers' wives, whoever they may be, telling them that I wasn't right about something I did. Therefore I hope that all of my family lives by what my parents teach us, because it does mean something.
>
> Family is a powerful word. It has a great deal of meaning behind it. You have certain feelings that are so much a part of your real self that can never be changed. Someone's attitudes can be changed by other people's actions or feelings, but your core self is very different. The relationship that I have with my family is a part of my core self and will always be a part of my core self. No matter who I marry, [that person] will never be able to know my family in the same way that I know them. Each person has his or her unique personality, and that is why my dad said for my brothers and my sister and me to keep the bond that we share now. My life with my family will always be what matters to me the most.

The more successful the shift in primary attachment from parents to mate, the greater the influence each person has over the other. The ideal developmental goal would be for couples to be open to the influence of others they respect while they form personal positions relatively free from emotional alignments. In practice however, this is more the exception than the rule. It's important therefore to sort out the potential sources of influence and how these competitive forces play themselves out in the triangles of marital conflict. Sometimes the influence of, say, one partner's parent is easy to see. Often the process is more subtle and difficult to ferret out. This process becomes overt at times in every marriage. Making wedding plans, choosing a place to live, buying a car, the birth of a baby, choosing a school, all are times when this struggle may become explicit. A classic example is the time of a birth, when a "battle of the grandmothers" may begin.

When Molly B. went into labor, she called her mother, who lived an hour away. Brad called his parents who lived even closer. The couple was well aware of what a major event a first grandchild was in close-knit Jewish families. The grandmothers-to-be each had had her own distinctive style—neither one was a shrinking violet. Molly wanted her mother to put the finishing touches on the baby's room, and Brad's mother had already headed for her local drugstore to make sure that there were plenty of diapers and other necessities on hand when the baby came home.

They named the baby Eli, after Brad's paternal grandfather. Molly's mother insisted that Eli have a middle name from their family. During Eli's first year Molly and Brad found themselves getting irritated with one another every time they discussed their parents. Until Eli's birth, the grandmothers hadn't been an issue, but Brad and Molly both felt that Eli's birth seemed to change things. The last straw had been when Molly's mother arrived 4 hours early for Eli's first birthday party, wanting to spend "alone" time with her grandson before Brad's parents arrived. The fact that the baby was napping and that Brad and Molly weren't ready for company didn't seem to faze her. A similar event had happened 2 weeks earlier when the families were supposed to get together to celebrate Fathers' Day. That time *Brad's* mother had dropped in so that she could be with Eli before the other Grandma got there.

In this case, the therapist coached each partner to work on the relationship with his or her own mother, making the shift from the child–parent relationship to the more functional adult–adult relationship. As Molly and Brad each spent more time one-on-one with their own mothers (without Eli), taking care to act like adults with them, the grandmothers' battle for Eli became less intense, and Molly and Brad got less reactive to it.

DISPLACEMENT OF CONFLICT

When problems with primacy of attachment and hierarchy of influence come up, a significant conflict may arise between a parent and a son- or daughter-in-law. Most often it represents unworked-out conflict between the parent and his or her own child, which gets displaced onto that child's mate. A familiar example is the husband who generously turns his mother over to his wife when he gets married. These men also implicitly and symbolically give their babies to their mothers. This is exemplified by the son who goes to his parents' house for a holiday meal and hands the baby over to his mother as he plops himself down in front of the television and avoids any personal conversation or discussion with her.

Another variant of this problem occurs when both spouses distance dramatically from conflictual or overcontrolling parents, seeking refuge from them in the marriage and creating a protective "cocoon" of their marriage. Both spouses do a frank or ritualized cutoff from their parents, keeping them at a distance, with the marriage serving as the refuge. In this situation, the emotional demands placed on the marriage are excessive, and the cocoon becomes oppressive. When a marriage such as this begins to fall apart (without an affair), people inevitably migrate back toward their family of origin. They then see their own family as a refuge from a "smothering" marriage. During a marriage all these stages may come into play at different times and in varying sequences. Thus the shifts can go back and forth from the primary parental triangle, to some variant of an in-law triangle, to an attempt at "cocooning."

We have considered the three major process factors that determine the mechanisms and forms of extended family triangles. Let us examine now each of the types and subtypes of these triangles.

IN-LAW TRIANGLES

When people pair off to create their own families, they need to shift their primary allegiance to the new relationship while they keep their connections to their original families. People function better in life if they maintain some kind of balance between the two families. The reason for keeping the balance is that it is less likely to set up the kind of circumstances that would demonize one family and idealize the other. The tendency is to cut off from the demonized side, and cutoffs are not functional as emotional processes. If the couple members don't consider their relationship with each other to be of primary importance, a variety of problems can result. The major reason for this is that the bond between the couple needs strengthening with history and connection so that it can withstand the pressures of life. On the other hand, the couple members also need to have strong relationship options within their families of origin so that all their emotional eggs are not in the one basket of their relationship.

Three subtypes of in-law triangles are particularly important in marital conflict: (1) the wedding gift triangle; (2) the loyalty alignment triangle; (3) the dominant father-in-law triangle. A therapist needs to figure out which specific form of in-law triangle is active at the time the case presents for treatment, work with the couple to identify and neutralize it, and eventually get back to the relevant material in each partner's primary parental triangle. The following guidelines may be useful:

1. Show through process questions and the therapist's own "I-positions" the importance of each spouse's taking responsibility for dealing with his or her own family.
2. Help the spouse least caught in an in-law triangle to experiment with detriangling maneuvers.
3. Work to increase the primacy of the marital bonding over that with parents.

The Wedding Gift Triangle

A culturally acceptable way for a man to avoid the pressure of a relationship with his mother without cutting her off is to hand her over to his wife. He gives her the responsibility of keeping in touch with his mother, seeing to it that his children have a relationship with her, buying gifts and birthday cards for her. In other words, a husband turns over to his wife the emotional or actual responsibility for his parents. After the wedding his mother becomes the wife's ally, or the wife's problem, or both, while the husband avoids real contact with his mother.

In this triangle, the husband's primacy of attachment is blurred and difficult to assess. Most often he assumes a distant position in relation to both his mother and his wife. The mother and wife have several ways they can deal with this dynamic. They may both like the idea and join together. They might form an alliance to shape up their distant son and husband, or they might simply bypass him, allowing him his distance and focus their energies on bringing up the children or even a joint business venture. In such cases, the wife is usually in flight from her family of origin, looking for membership and a sense of belonging in a new and different clan.

When this triangle presents clinically as marital conflict, it usually takes the form of a dysfunction in the husband. For example, he may be involved in an affair or may be abusing alcohol. The process in this triangle has the husband feeling relieved at first by the connection between his wife and mother. As time passes, however, even *his* tolerance for being on the outside is exceeded. Relief turns into feelings of rejection and lack of being appreciated. Explicit attempts by both wife and mother to shape him up with abundant criticism and emotionality sometimes reinforce these feelings. That is when the husband ends up absorbing the concern and anxiety of both wife and mother, and his functioning declines. He may turn to alcohol abuse or seek refuge in an extramarital affair to calm his inner turmoil.

The clinical management of this triangle calls for the therapist, having made an adequate connection with the wife, to encourage her to experiment one at a time with the following moves: (1) separate herself from her overinvolvement with her mother-in-law; (2) decrease her efforts at managing her husband; (3) look to her functioning as a wife rather than as mother and daughter-in-law; and (4) investigate the way her position in her primary parental triangle played a part in setting her up for her present position in the in-law triangle with her husband and his mother. Frequently in this situation, the wife has cut herself off from a primary parental triangle in which her father may have been an alcoholic and her mother dominant and controlling.

The husband must concentrate on mastering his dysfunction. If it's alcohol abuse, he must do whatever it takes to get control of his drinking; if it's an occupational dysfunction, he needs to work on getting a job. In time the therapist will encourage him to assume more responsibility for dealing with his own mother. He will also have to sort out the emotional factors that trigger him to take a position of extreme distance in relation to his wife and mother.

A variant on this pattern is the one in which the wife is depressed, with her husband and her mother united in criticism of her. Husband and his mother-in-law may not otherwise be close, and their only unity may be in their attempt to "shape up" wife/daughter. Nevertheless, the closer their relationship is, the worse it is for the wife. The clinical management of this variation is similar to the first: The husband must disengage from his alliance with his mother-in-law and stop his criticism of his wife; the underfunctioning wife needs to manage her own dysfunction, whatever it is, and then take on her own parent.

It is a basic principle that the responsibility for tending the relationship in their own families of origin belongs to the biological offspring.

More common than the situation we have just discussed is the mother-in-law and daughter-in-law who both rebel against the attempted relationship graft. In this situation, the unresolved emotional struggle between mother and son is displaced into a sometimes open, sometimes camouflaged, conflict between his mother and his wife. The underlying issue is usually the question of who has more influence and control over the husband.

Kim and Henry A., a couple in their mid-30s, were in conflict. Kim was overwrought because Henry had been disappearing for many hours at a time, and she had no idea where he was or what he was doing. On further exploration, Henry described his need to "get out of the house" at times. He had a vague idea that it was related to stress. He found his wife to be extremely intense, although he liked her warmth. Kim and he fought, usually at Kim's provocation, over Henry's mother. Henry didn't understand why Kim was so critical of his mother, although Henry admitted he rarely saw her himself, and when he spoke to her it was very superficially. Kim resented Henry's mother's continual intrusion into her life, with daily phone calls and questions about Henry and the children. Often she was critical of Kim and gave her unsolicited advice. Kim also resented Henry's lack of sympathy toward her when she complained about his mother. He pleaded with the therapist to get Kim to stop being so negative and upset about his mother.

It was clear to the therapist that Henry had handed his mother over to Kim since the beginning of the marriage and had allowed himself to continue to distance from his mother. As an adolescent, Henry ran from his mother. She had been an anxious, overprotective woman who could not allow her son privacy. She wouldn't allow Henry to close his bedroom door, and at times she would go through his drawers. As an adolescent, he of course had found this to be an intolerable intrusion. He had never said anything to his mother because he saw her as a "hysterical type of woman," and he didn't want to upset her. Henry's father had always been careful either to agree with his wife or to keep quiet. Henry had reacted to her invasion by distancing to such a degree that he had stayed as far from her as he could. Once, for example, when he found his mother going through his dresser drawers, Henry had left the house and was gone for 2 days, whereabouts unknown. Rather than deal with her, he had disappeared in much the same way he had been handling his reactivity to Kim.

The therapist first focused on Kim's extreme emotionality. She was crying a lot and not sleeping. She was so distressed about her mother-in-law that she turned red in the face when speaking of her. She was interested in calming her reactivity to her mother-in-law when the therapist explained that one day she might be a mother-in-law herself, and she could avoid this trap if she had a handle on her own situation. She also loved the idea that Henry needed to take more responsibility for his mother.

First Kim was coached to stop expecting some kind of abstract, ideal in-law relationship. The therapist suggested that she begin calling her mother-in-law to ask for her advice rather than trying to escape her phone calls. She was also coached to take more initiative in saying no to her mother-in-law. When questions came up about Henry, Kim directed her to her son. Kim also was directed to talk to her own mother about her mother's difficult relationship with Kim's paternal grandmother. This work helped Kim see the three-generational issues in her own family of origin and their effect on her marriage. When the therapist taught Kim how to handle her mother-in-law differently, Kim calmed down. Now, the therapy could turn toward encouraging Henry to take on the project of dealing with his mother and to work on his running from the pressure he feels when faced with two women who want to have a relationship with him. Kim was encouraged to review her response when she felt Henry's distance.

In a case like Kim and Henry's, until the husband accepts responsibility for dealing with his mother and their relationship, and until the wife accepts responsibility for giving him the freedom to do it, the potential for trouble in the relationship remains high. Clinically, this goal can be achieved by helping the husband to accept this responsibility directly or by coaching the wife to lower her reactivity and use her creativity indirectly and subtly to create a climate that gives the husband and his mother the best chance for a successful relationship.

The Loyalty Alignment Triangle

In the loyalty alignment triangle, a partner and his or her parent (or other family member) remain overly close, with the other partner in the distant position. This triangle occurs when one or both partners never really leave their family of origin.

When a therapist asked one wife how she got so bitter toward her husband of 23 years, she replied, "It was the night before our wedding. We had just made love. I looked at John and asked, 'Who do you love more, me or your mother?' He said, 'My mother, of course!' I never forgave him."

The loyalty alignment triangle centers on primacy of attachment and hierarchy of influence. One spouse, perhaps the husband, is in an overly close relationship with his family of origin. His wife is in the outside position, unable to get the kind of membership she is looking for in her husband's family or, what is more important, the bond she wants with him. When a conflictual or toxic issue arises, such as money, the people who have the most influence over the husband may still be his family, especially his mother. Thus does the influence of the extended family and attachment to it take precedence over the marital relationship.

The planning of the wedding itself can provide the trigger for the loyalty alignment triangle to be set in motion. Such was the case for Beth and David A., a couple in their early 20s. They called the therapist 5 weeks before the wedding. Beth had broken the engagement after a scene between David and her that occurred after they had been with her mother. The topic of contention was table cloths. Beth and her mother wanted black tablecloths at the wedding reception, while David thought that black was too depressing a color for a wedding. His grandmother, with whom he had been very close, had died recently, and he cited this as a reason against black.

As David told the therapist, "I really like Beth's mother, but I feel like it's not our wedding; it's Beth's and her mother's." Beth explained that all her life she and her mother had planned and talked about her wedding day. She didn't think David had a right to interfere with her mother's dreams. "After all, my parents *are* paying for the wedding." This triangle shows the real difficulty this young woman had in shifting her loyalty to her husband-to-be. Although David protested that he liked his mother-in-law-to-be, it wouldn't be a surprise to find that he would soon learn to resent her.

In this situation, the therapist chose to do some education of David and Beth. She explained the importance of forming a dyad as they enter this new stage of life while finding a way to keep a connection with their families of origin. The therapist discussed the many situations that might occur as this young couple went about the events that surrounded their wedding. She pointed out that, although they were concerned with tablecloth color, they faced a dilemma that was classic and that needed sensitive handling. Beth and her mother were going through an emotional time. Beth was encouraged to focus on her mother's feelings about the change in Beth's status in the family from daughter to David's wife. What would that mean for the relationship between Beth and her mother? How was Beth going to have a woman-to-woman relationship with her mother? The therapist also did some talking with David about his sadness that his grandmother was no longer alive to be part of his wedding. When Beth understood that black made David too sad, and that it was not an anti-Beth's-mother decision, she was quite willing to change the table-cloth color to something less funereal. She also explained to her mother that David's feelings were important to her. David was immediately relieved. He felt that he was now number one on Beth's list of priorities. The wedding went off without a hitch.

The Dominant Father-in-Law Triangle

In the dominant father-in-law triangle, a wife and her idealized father are united in implicit criticism of the husband. This triangle can be significant in marital conflict even when the wife's father is dead. Olivia C., a 44-year-old nurse, complained about a depression in her daughter, Justine, whose boyfriend had been in trouble with the law and had run away from home. Olivia's husband, Kyle, was a distant, angry father, and there was much conflict in the family, especially between Olivia and Kyle. Kyle was essentially uninvolved with Justine. Olivia's father had been a much-revered, dominant man. He was an attorney on a pedestal of his own making and adored by his daughter. Olivia silently and not so silently compared her husband with her father and found her husband wanting. Kyle resented Olivia's attachment to her father and her preoccupation with their daughter. He displayed this anger by his passive distance from the daughter.

Three interlocking triangles were present. One had Kyle in a distant position, with Olivia and Justine overly close. In another, Kyle was in the distant position, with Olivia and her father overly close. A third triangle had Olivia and her father overly close, with Olivia's mother in the distant position. These triangles functioned to stabilize all the twosomes in the marriages of both generations by involving a third person, namely a child. Activators included any attempt by one marital partner to modify the closeness–distance relationship in the two marriages. The process, once started, took the form of one parent feeling excluded by the other parent and convinced that the other parent is giving to a child the sympathy, interest, and attention wanted by the first parent. The parent–child over closeness was perpetuated from one generation to another, and it interfered with the marriage of the involved child. This gave the father-in-law an unholy influence over the next generation.

Intervening meant narrowing the distances and distancing the over closenesses so that everyone moved toward a more balanced position. This involved showing Olivia a way that made sense to her to be less involved with Justine and to leave Justine room to develop a real relationship with her father. A dilemma for the therapist usually arises at this point: How do you make the shifting of positions in a triangle relevant to the family? Suppose Olivia had said, "Hey, if Kyle were a better father, I wouldn't have any need to be in there with Justine as much as I am!" She'd have a point. One way to deal with objections like that one is to remind the person in Olivia's position that she is her daughter's role model for how to deal with men. She is also modeling how to deal with other relationships, like the one between Olivia and her own mother. You can remind her that what her daughter learns may be what she can expect between Justine and herself in years to come. Making it worthwhile for Olivia to change what she does in the family and to see the positive by-products for her self and her daughter down the road often inspires an interest in change.

Olivia needed considerable coaching around her level of criticism toward Kyle as she pulled back from Justine because she would be leaving a vacuum that Kyle may (or may not) move in to fill. If he does, it would not be in the way that Olivia would think is adequate. The therapist reminded Olivia of several things to think about that would help her through the transition. First, she should expect to be anxious as she moves away. She should stay focused on what is occurring inside her rather than looking at what is going on with the other two legs of the triangle (Kyle and Justine). Second, one can't simply move away from one anchor toward nothing. That won't work. Olivia needed to concentrate on another important project. The project here was narrowing the distance in her relationship with her mother and lowering her reactivity to her mother. The therapist pointed out to Olivia that she and her mother had a relationship similar to that between Kyle and Justine. Encouraging her to alter this pattern made the shift make sense to Olivia. Letting her know that Justine might benefit made her more enthusiastic.

Third, the therapist explained to Kyle and Olivia that Kyle

needed practice in exercising his relationship muscles with Justine, since they had atrophied from lack of use. The therapist also made it explicit that mistakes were inevitable *and allowed.* This gave the couple a powerful message—that the direction of movement is more important than the nature of the movement. It is more important that Kyle be moving toward Justine than that every move be perfect. Kyle had hung back from Justine perhaps partly due to a lack of confidence in his parenting or perhaps because he thought Olivia as a woman was better equipped to handle Justine. He would probably feel awkward and unsure once he started to become a more active parent. The therapist helped him by gently encouraging his attempts to get to know his daughter in his own style. Meanwhile, the therapist helped Olivia in getting to know her mother as a woman by suggesting, for instance, that two women who have daughters could have an interesting conversation.

Fourth, the therapist taught Olivia and Kyle to monitor their anxiety as they began to shift the triangular pattern. This is a good way to lead people toward the next therapeutic intervention: learning self-focus and about what internal pressures fuel their movement in relationships. The therapist knew that marital issues might surface during this work, and the more willing and Olivia and Kyle were to focus on their own parts in their problems, the more accessible the marital issues would be to intervention.

This case is a good example of how the proper handling of an extended family triangle (here, the dominant father-in-law triangle) has positive effects on nuclear family relationships. By altering the movement in that triangle, Olivia and Kyle helped their child and made work on their marriage possible.

Spouse and Spouse's Sibling Triangles

Nancy G., a 42-year-old, perfectly dressed woman, had no trouble telling the therapist what she thought the major source of difficulty was in her marriage: her selfish and lazy sisters-in-law, whom her husband, Frank, treated like princesses. She let him know plainly that she disapproved of them and of his behavior toward them. Frank's response was to lose his temper and call Nancy names. The couple had a history of conflict in their relationship, often ending with Frank swearing at Nancy and putting her down. As for Nancy, she had no problems other than Frank with his family.

Frank, a successful and wealthy corporate executive, confessed that Nancy was right. He got frustrated and hopeless about their marriage because Nancy wasn't affectionate and didn't talk much. He also said with a laugh that her hobby was spending money. Nancy's reaction to that kind of comment was predictable: She would get red in the face and vehemently defend herself.

The most recent explosion concerned the fighting going on over an upcoming Passover seder. Every holiday both extended families congregated at Nancy and Frank's house. Nancy was furious because Frank's sisters, as usual, "never lifted a finger" to help her, nor did they "ever offer to bring anything." Nancy was sick of it. So this year she refused to do anything in preparation. She was on strike. Frank, on the other hand, defended his sisters and pointedly criticized Nancy for a lack of domestic abilities. Moreover, he resented Nancy's continual litany of negative comments about his sisters. He agreed that they weren't the most helpful of women—but they were, after all, *his* sisters. The holiday issue was not the only one Nancy said frosted her about Frank and his sisters. "Besides being lazy, they are money-grubbing. Frank doles out money, sometimes exorbitant amounts, every time they turn around. Not only that, he sees nothing wrong with it. If he gives them $10,000, he should give me $10,000, but he doesn't!" The clinical trap here is that almost everyone, from casual observer to experienced therapist is likely to agree with Nancy's compelling logic about these gifts to Frank's sisters. There's no doubt that Frank was arbitrary in giving substantial sums to his sisters without consulting Nancy, his life partner. The point, however, is that this dispute needed to be focused on, not in terms of its content, but in terms of the triangular structure and process that it so beautifully illustrated. As we'll see below, that's how the therapist dealt with it.

Frank and Nancy have been married for 24 years. They grew up in the same town and lived around the corner from one another. Nancy was the older of two children. She and her younger brother were distant, and she said that she didn't like him. She described her parents' marriage as horrible and her childhood as very unhappy. Her father spent no time with her mother, and, although he made a comfortable living, he never spent any of it on his wife or children. Nancy said that her father had always disliked her and let her know that in every possible way. She described him with no emotion and didn't seem to think his coldness was a big deal. Her relationship with her mother was conflictual, although they had daily contact, usually over the phone.

Frank described his family as "your normal, happy family." Nancy interrupted with a different picture, in which the family had overindulged the daughters and had treated Frank, the only boy, more harshly. Frank was the oldest of the three children. His sisters were quite dependent on him as an adviser and for money. At the time the couple came to therapy, Frank was supporting both sisters. The older was married, and her husband was in legal and financial trouble. Frank had purchased their home, and although the money was a loan, Nancy was skeptical that they would ever repay it. The other sister didn't work, and Frank had supported her for several years.

Frank had become the head of his family at age 21 when his father died suddenly. This had been a tremendous shock for him, and it had devastated the family. To this day, Frank sees it as his responsibility to take care of his mother and sisters.

As a boy, Frank had been very dependent on his mother, according to him. He had difficulty leaving her even to go to college, and even now he has anxiety about taking trips and leaving home. Frank's relationship with his mother had changed dramatically since his father died. Now he was taking care of her.

Frank and Nancy had a son and a daughter. The daughter was 22 and had been diagnosed with a seizure disorder since early adolescence. Although she had graduated recently from college, her seizures have remained hard to control. Their son is apparently without problems. Both Frank and Nancy think their daughter is doing well, considering the nature of her difficulties, and deny any problems with her. Frank is, however, quick to say that Nancy is not warm enough to the children.

The triangle that brought Nancy and Frank to therapy was highly fixed. Frank and his sisters were very involved, and Nancy was in the outside position. Most of the time this triangle wasn't apparent, and when the couple were getting along you wouldn't have known that it existed. However, when a holiday was on the horizon, with Nancy obligated to provide food and hospitality to Frank's family, or when Nancy learned that Frank had given money to either of his sisters, the triangle became explicit and active.

There was little fluidity in this triangle. The distances among all three participants were static. Nancy was explicitly or implicitly negative about Frank's sisters, moving neither closer to nor further away from them. Frank was always defensive about his sisters and irritated at Nancy's attitude toward them. The triangle was rigid, fixed, and chronic. The predictable nature of the participants' responses is the clue to the triangle's rigidity.

The problems that this triangle raised for the couple needed to be made relevant to their original problem. It wasn't difficult here since Nancy was aware that the fighting and her anger about Frank's sisters had been going on since they were married. Frank acknowledged that he had no sympathy for Nancy's attitude. The therapist knew from experience that the relationship difficulties between Frank and Nancy were "safer" coming out around the issue of the sisters than in another area. She tested that assumption by doing the following.

First, she calmed down the conflict by suggesting that Nancy change her position in the triangle. She urged no more criticism or complaining to Frank about his family. The therapist's expectation was that, if Nancy began to act less reactively in the triangle, she would eventually be less reactive.

Second, she asked that Frank take responsibility for helping Nancy with the holiday celebration and for having the children help Nancy.

Third, Frank was asked to delegate food assignments to his sisters.

Fourth, the therapist explored the issue of money. She discovered that Nancy was more upset about the unequal treatment she was getting from her husband than about his not giving her money. In fact, Nancy thought he was very generous toward her and the children. Though he put her down for her spending, he never limited her. Nancy also felt independent, since she earned some money as a real estate agent.

Fifth, the therapist took a position with Nancy that she was out of line fighting with Frank over whether he gave his sisters money. A more important driving force lay beneath her anger. It concerned how much influence she felt his sisters and his mother had with him, compared to how much influence Nancy had with him. The therapist discussed the disparity in power in the context of Frank's responsibility to his mother and sisters since his father's death and Nancy not feeling that *she* was his number-one priority.

With both spouses making their assigned changes in the triangle, the conflict became less of an issue for the moment. What took its place was another triangle. The couple shifted their conflict to the issue of their son, Alan, whom they had originally described as "doing just fine." Alan had left home for his first year in college, and he was miserable. Both parents were anxious but were in conflict about how to handle the problem. The same issues came up again: Nancy's coldness and Frank's nastiness toward her.

It was at this point that the couple began to see that the external difficulties that cause the conflict between them are only a piece of the emotional process that they needed to address. They began to see the real question as this: What is it, in the nature of the dyad and in themselves as individuals, that is causing the dysfunction between them? The use of triangles as a treatment structure was extremely useful in getting the couple to this point. It was also useful in avoiding therapy being bogged down in arbitration about money and holidays.

Nancy and Frank have maintained the progress they made in therapy. In a recent letter to the therapist, Nancy reported that, "in spite of some surprises"—a promotion for Frank and Alice's engagement to the boy they had hoped she would never marry—they are working hard *together* to be happy. Frank built their dream house, Nancy decorated the inside and Frank the outside, and both are happy with the way it turned out. They are 1 year out of therapy.

Clinical Management of In-Law Triangles

If the therapist and couple's plan is to work on the issues in the couple's relationship for an open-ended period, they can probably address most of the triangles mentioned here. If the number of sessions is limited (e.g., by managed care), the therapist should concentrate on the following:

1. To start with the most proximate, symptomatic triangle, and work through eventually to each spouse's primary parental triangle.
2. To set up an increasing primacy of the marital bond without doing damage to the relationships the spouses have with their parents.
3. To help the spouses in developing an ability to sort out the sources of influence on them and be able to arrive at their own positions and courses of action without alienating important others.
4. To shift displaced conflict and bitterness to the appropriate relationship context, and to deal with it there.

THE PRIMARY PARENTAL TRIANGLE OF EACH SPOUSE

Invariably, the place each partner has occupied in his or her original family will have significant impact on the marital conflict. This is par-

ticularly true of the process involving each person in the primary parental triangle (the triangle consisting of him or herself and his or her
parents). That triangle is the basic training ground for each spouse's
emotional maturity. We can measure the emotional maturity of each
spouse largely by the degree to which each of them can operate
within that primary parental triangle with a low amount of anxiety. It
is also a measure of how much of each of them is emotionally available for bonding in the marital relationship.

For example, the more a husband is expending psychic energy
fending off or giving in to the implicit and explicit emotional demands of his mother, the less he is available for forming a primary attachment with his wife. Furthermore, if he cuts off from his mother,
he repeats the problems with her in his relationship with his wife.
This is not to say that "he marries his mother" but that he has been
sensitized to emotional issues left unresolved between his mother and
him. Remember the case of Henry and Kim (pp. 175–176). He hadn't
married his mother—Kim was very different from her mother-in-law.
What *was* similar was the anxiety that Henry experienced when he
was faced with Kim's expression of emotions, especially if he had
caused them. His automatic emotional response was to shut up and
head for the hills. On a good day he was defensive. Thus, the primary
parental triangle is the training ground for all other relationships. If
people can learn to desensitize their knee-jerk reactions to certain behaviors and attitudes in their parents, the other relationships in their
lives will be flow more easily. The same is true for psychotherapists
who are interested in learning how to manage their emotional triggers in couple therapy. The secret is to manage people's reactivity in
getting to know their parents.

The reactive process in one's primary parental triangle influences
the marital relationship in at least two other ways. First, it presensitizes
the individual to certain emotional triggers that set off an automatic internal emotional response and subsequent reactive behavior. The best
example of this is the case in which one spouse comes from a family with
alcohol abuse. That spouse has been sensitized to alcohol as an issue
and often to a particular form of drunken comportment as well. Second, it sets up patterns of compliance and submissiveness or the opposite patterns of counter-positioning and revolution.

We can illustrate two interesting variants on the latter phenomenon. Imagine a wife's special relationship with her father, a prominent and successful man. If her mother's response to this special relationship had been to pressure and criticize her, one response might

be to rebel openly against her mother. Her rebellion would come from the strength gained from her relationship with her father and even, perhaps, with his covert support. She would then be more likely to approach a conflict with her husband by openly challenging him and threatening revolution if he did not accept her terms or stop his undesirable behavior.

Let's change the scenario just a little, making the wife's father only marginally successful and submissive to his wife in their relationship. Then, her mother's pressure and criticism might produce submissive, compliant behavior from the wife. In her marriage, when her husband and her mother join forces to shape her up, she is a set-up for becoming adaptive and subsequently dysfunctional. Here her dysfunction becomes her only source of leverage in the system.

There are three goals in working in the primary parental triangle of one or both spouses:

1. Discover and make explicit the way that the primary parental triangle of each partner is relevant to the emotional process in the marriage. For example, both partners may have clung to each other from early in the relationship as a way of escaping the conflict or the stickiness of inordinate attachment. Likewise, one partner may be overly distant or cut off from his family, while the other partner remains overly attached to hers. Each of these configurations puts extra pressure on the developing marital relationship.

2. Coach both spouses to increase their ability to operate nonreactively within their own primary parental triangles. This is a laudable goal in theory, but in clinical reality, one partner is usually much more motivated than the other to do extended family work. At any rate, it is important for the therapist to foster a respect and sensitivity in each partner for the position of the other in this matter. As one woman put it, "If you're not going to work on your family, at least don't undermine me working on mine."

3. Help each spouse to sort out his or her bitterness, by differentiating between the bitterness that truly comes from the spouse and that which comes from the primary parental triangle.

The therapist must get a clear picture of each spouse's primary parental triangle in the evaluation of every marital conflict. We accomplish this most easily and efficiently while taking the genogram. Working with each spouse in the primary parental triangle can best be seen as individual work within marital therapy. We spoke at length about this process when we talked about the primary parental triangle in dealing with individuals.[1]

TRIANGLES WITH THE CHILDREN

A couple's children are ready-made for a triangle. It would be difficult to imagine a more convenient way of confusing issues or diluting tension between husband and wife than by triangling in one or more of their children. From the moment of conception, a child is a potential third person in a triangle. Chapters 11 and 12 are devoted to triangles in which children are caught, but seeing how children can be in the middle of a marital case is important. Vito and Fran M. are such a case. They were both raised in Italian-American families, and their relationships with their mothers have enormous impact on their marriage.

Vito and Fran came to therapy in the middle of a crisis that had been going on for several weeks. Vito had lost 15 pounds in the prior 2 weeks and hadn't been sleeping. Fran took full responsibility for the difficulty. She told the therapist that Vito had hired a detective and had tapped their phone. He found out that she had been seeing Sam, a colleague at work. She denied anything sexual but admitted, "Sure, I like him." She cried and said that she was an outsider in her own house. She looked at the floor all the time she was speaking. Vito, also crying, declared that "the worst part of this is what she's doing to our girls."

Vito and Fran had two daughters, 17 and 12. The older was obviously Vito's special child; he spoke sympathetically of her anger at her mother for abandoning everyone. Fran's behavior was no secret from the children, and her mother was calling the house daily, knowing that something was wrong. Vito had briefed his mother-in-law on Fran's transgressions and had told his own family, his mother and sister in particular.

When taking a history, the therapist became interested in the longstanding problems between Fran and her older daughter. Vito had always appropriated Fran's role with her daughter, and she had never done anything about it because she was afraid he would misunderstand her. "Every child should have an involved father," she would say. She described how strange it felt not to have a connection with

---

[1]See Chapters 7 and 8.

her own child, especially because she was so close to her own mother. In fact, she admitted, she was so close to her mother that sometimes she almost couldn't breathe. Her mother had to know everything that went on in her and Vito's lives. If she didn't learn it from Fran, she got it from Vito. Fran said that it had been like that all her life. When asked where her father was, she replied that he had been "out doing his thing."

When Fran and Vito became more comfortable with therapy and had calmed down a bit, the therapist learned that the younger daughter had been coming into bed with them almost every night since their marriage had blown up. Fran explained that both kids hung out in the bedroom, and the 12-year-old had been sleeping off and on in their room since she had been born.

Vito described his parents as similar to Fran's. His father had been busy at work 7 days a week, and his mother, whom he described as crazy and cruel, had abused his older brother physically. Vito had become a well-behaved little boy once he figured out that then his mother wouldn't hit him. He had looked to his older sister for nurturance and made it his business to avoid his mother. (He still makes it his business to avoid her.)

It's easy to see how Vito and Fran's marriage had been vulnerable to involving the children in their problems. They hadn't dealt with separating from their own parents. They had followed their parents' pattern by not dealing with each other and including the children where they didn't belong. Before this couple could turn things around in their marriage, Fran had to end the extramarital triangle, and both had to place appropriate boundaries between themselves and their daughters. They also had to address their primary parental triangles and the triangles with each child.

The two major functions served by triangles with the children in marital conflict are covering over the marital conflict and letting parenting become the issue around which partners organize their marital conflict. The ways these triangles can work are many, and families play innumerable variations on the theme. These triangles overlap with the nuclear family subtypes of child and adolescent intrafamilial triangles, considered below.

A common pattern in couples that present with marital conflict is a parent in the overly close and defensive position with a child, and the spouse in the distant and critical position. The criticism can be directed either at the child, or the other parent, or both. Ruth and Gil E. are an example. They had two children, of whom the older, Zach, was 5 years old and had a chronic illness. Gil told the therapist that he was furious with Ruth because she waited on the child hand and foot, indulging his most ludicrous demands. It was so bad that it now took Zach an hour to get dressed before school because he changed his clothes five or six times. Moreover, Ruth was carrying Zach around like a baby. Ruth explained how scary Gil was when he was angry, and how much he frightened Zach. Ruth believed that Zach was behaving like this because of Gil. When the therapist explored the couple's history, it became evident that underneath this very hot triangle was a severe sexual problem. Gil felt deprived in the sexual relationship because Ruth had no interest in being sexually intimate. It had been several years according to both spouses since they had enjoyed sexual contact.

The questions of primacy of attachment (Who is your number-one relationship?) and hierarchy of influence (Whom are you going to listen to?) are issues that married people often raise with each other in one form or another: "Whom are you married to, me or your mother?" "Your father doesn't make the decisions in this house." "I was here before your precious daughter." With an eye on these two themes, this chapter has reviewed the key intrafamilial triangles that complicate the marital relationship. We turn now to a closer examination of triangles that have children and adolescents at their center.

CHAPTER ELEVEN

Child and Adolescent Triangles

The notion of child- and adolescent-centered triangles in the family began in the late 1950s, and received considerable clinical attention in the 1960s and 1970s. Today therapists across the board almost universally accept these triangles as a clinically significant phenomenon. Since Guerin and Gordon's work on the typology of child and adolescent triangles,[1] we remain convinced that their typology is a useful tool for the clinician to see the way relationship processes feed into the development of symptoms in children and adolescents. There are seven categories in our version of the typology. We discuss them in this chapter and the next.

SCHOOL-RELATED TRIANGLES

A common presentation in child-centered families is a symptomatic child whose primary symptom involves misbehavior or relationship conflict at school, or refusal to go to school ("school phobia"). As is always the case in child-centered families, symptom relief is therapy's first priority. Without symptom relief, you have no credibility with a child-centered family. The second priority, if the family is interested, is dealing with the system-wide difficulties that triggered or main-

---

[1]Guerin and Gordon (1986).

tained the symptom. It will not surprise the reader to learn that both these goals require the discovery and neutralization of the triangles that are active in these cases.

A school-related problem usually involves one or more of the following five factors:

1. The symptomatic child is often the most emotionally vulnerable member of the family, and this vulnerability is being played out in school rather than within the family.
2. An explicit conflict is going on between the symptomatic child and a school authority figure, usually the teacher.
3. A covert conflict between the child and one or both of the parents is being displaced into the relationship between the child and the teacher.
4. The symptomatic child has a special relationship with the teacher that makes the child a target of some less favored powerful students in the classroom.
5. The child is caught up in a triangle based on a conflict, explicit or covert, between a parent and the teacher.[2]

The first task for the therapist, therefore, is diagnostic. Sometimes, the school-related problem may be a displacement of a family problem. Here, the key triangle is an *intrafamilial* one such as the target child triangle[3] or a parent–sibling triangle. The child may be playing out his or her part in the marital problems at home or in sibling rivalry triangles from the family, and continuing this process in school. An extrafamiliar triangle may also be present, with teacher, principal, or fellow student bringing their own triangles into the problem. These alternatives may be difficult to sort out and, in fact, may be coexistent. In all these situations, the proof is in the pudding. If the teacher can go one-on-one with the student and the parents can do the same thing, then a triangle isn't active. If the parties involved don't repeat the patterns over and over again, a triangle isn't active. However, if a parent or teacher continues to see the circumstances in the same way and avoids looking at his or her own part in the problem, that shows where the triangle is active. Over time, the fixity of the process and the predictability of responses place the triangle in the family, the school, or both. The advantage of formulating the

---

[2]Guerin and Katz (1984).

[3]See discussion on "the target child" in Chapter 12.

problem about the family is that it gives much more control to the family. It allows the father to work on himself and his part in the problem and the same for mother and child. This is easier and more "doable" than trying to change the school system.

The therapist should not assume, however, that every school problem is merely a displacement of an intrafamilial problem. Frequently, the active triangle involves the child, a parent, and a teacher or other school figure. In its most common form, the parent–child–teacher triangle is the result of a displacement of a parent–child conflict to the teacher–child relationship. A dramatic difference between the child's home and school behavior often marks this process. The reactivity of the child to the parent, usually around the issues of control and authority, comes out in school. If the involved parent and teacher join forces to "shape up" the child, the problem behavior escalates. The most effective way of intervening in such a situation is to encourage the uninvolved parent to take over the functions of parenting, including dealing with the school and the teacher.

Some people believe that problems at home result from enmeshed permissive parenting, whereas problems at school result from enmeshed strict parenting. We may sometimes see this connection, but such formulations go beyond our current knowledge. Acting out at school may come from strictness at home, permissiveness at home, and from some disability—emotional, biological, or characterological—in the individual child. To avoid falling into a blaming triangle, we therapists need to remember that the "best" of parents may have a child who acts out at school.

In another form of the parent–child–teacher triangle, the parent has a conflict with the teacher, perhaps because of a personality clash or because of a disagreement about educational methods. The child acts out the parent's feelings toward the teacher. This is a common variation when the parent is a professional, especially a teacher. Again, the appropriate intervention is to ask the uninvolved parent to take over dealings with the teacher and the school. Remember that the family is only one form of system. The members of all groups are related in some form of systematic process, and often these systems function with different purposes, even at cross-purposes. All systems seek inner balance and survival (self-perpetuation). With the breakdown in family systems and the intact family, society has shifted ever more responsibility for the child to the community and, in particular, to the school. This has often given the school responsibility without authority—a sure prescription for trouble.

Sometimes the triangle is activated because the child triggers an emotional reaction in the teacher—a reaction triggered by another aspect of the teacher's life. In this situation, the parent shouldn't join too readily with the teacher in her or his criticism of the child. If the parent does so, we may miss the teacher's part in the problem, and the problem behavior will escalate. Sometimes, involving the school's administration to help the teacher in seeing the emotional trigger is necessary to resolve this kind of problem.

Chris J. was an 11-year-old boy with problems at school. He had few friends, was picked on by older children, and mostly he was isolated or spent time with adults. His school-related problems began when he started kindergarten, during which his mother had described him as "psychosomatic" and "school phobic." Chris's special needs as a young child had complicated these symptoms; a hip deformity had temporarily made him an invalid. Chris's mother had always been very involved with Chris and his school problems, and she had been the primary caregiver when he wore braces to correct his physical disability. His father had usually been in the distant position. Chris and his mother had been seen for 18 months in individual therapy at a local child guidance clinic. The father had not been involved in the treatment.

A series of nodal events had coincided to create sufficient stress to begin the triangulation process in several interlocking triangles fixed for the past 12 years. During Chris's first year of life, Mrs. J.'s father had died. She and 10-month-old Chris remained in England while Mr. J. relocated to the United States, where Chris and his mother joined him 6 months later. When Chris was 6 and starting first grade, Mrs. J. had reason to be seriously concerned about her mother's health. Chris, alert to his mother's upset about her extended family in England, became symptomatic. The outbreak of Chris's symptoms coincided with the covert marital conflict about parental responsibility. This pattern had continued to recycle and turned out to be the context in which Chris's therapist sought a consultation about Chris's refusal to go to school.

A symptomatic child caught in a conflict with a teacher is often displacing his anxiety about conflict between his parents, stress in the extended family, or both. The conflict with the teacher may be explicit or implicit. In Chris's case, the conflict is implicit, and took the form of his refusal to go to school. When this symptom had first appeared, many factors combined to form a very stressful context and to activate several triangles: the intergenerational triangle in which Chris, sensitized when he was an infant to stress in his mother's family, triangled with his mother and her concerns about her own mother's health; and the primary parental triangle, activated by the marital conflict around parenting issues.

By the time Chris and his mother were seen in consultation, the school-related triangle was the immediate problem. It had to be dealt with before the underlying, intrafamilial issues and triangles could be dealt with. Mrs. J.'s response to Chris's school problems had been to increase the focus on him by pressuring him about going to school. She also pressured the school to get more services for him and to transfer him to another school. The consultant recommended to the therapist that Mrs. J. be coached to pull back from pressuring Chris or the school. He suggested that she learn to monitor her reactions to this move and bring those reactions into therapy. Finally, the marital and extended family issues would inevitably become explicit if Mrs. J. was no longer displacing them onto Chris and the school. At that point Mrs. J. should involve Mr. J. in the treatment and move to the underlying issues of parenting responsibilities and extended family concerns.

SOCIAL NETWORK TRIANGLES

As adolescents turn their loyalties away from their parents and toward their friends (or, if you prefer the fancier term, their "peer network"), it's inevitable that certain potential triangles will be activated. The structural pattern in these triangles is consistent. The parents are in the outside distant position with the adolescent and influential friends locked in a generationally protective alliance.

Just about everyone (unless she or he is the parent involved) knows that such a setup is developmentally appropriate and, within reason, fosters normal development in all parties involved. The adolescent invests emotionally in an object other than a parent. This chosen friend becomes one of the adolescent's "transitional objects"—the teenage equivalent of the child's teddy bear. The parent gets to experience the beginnings of a lifetime of losing influence and letting go, while always being on emotional call—and expected to like it. This normal developmental process becomes symptomatic when it is polarized by external or internal stress on one or all of the parties that make up this relationship triangle. The following example may help to clarify these points.

Dana W. was a 13-year-old, the younger of two siblings; her older brother, Fred, was 16. Mr. W. was an overworked, highly successful attorney, home only on weekends, and some weeks not at all. Mrs. W. worked part-time in her own consulting business and focused most of her parenting attention on her son. Dana resented this, but she also found the benign neglect liberating. Besides, she knew that her father thought of her as special. In addition, during the year before coming to therapy she had formed an intense attachment to Sabrina, a new classmate who had recently moved into their neighborhood from (where else?) California. Dana was not only enamored of Sabrina, but also thought that Sabrina's mother was "really cool." Sabrina was a good student, an excellent tennis player, and very facile with adults. She also had a compulsion for shopping malls and for the guys who frequent them. Sabrina's mother thought this precocious sexuality was cute.

Dana's mother had brought her to the clinic for evaluation after an incident in which Dana had been sent to her room as punishment for an intensely negative, prolonged, and profane outburst. She had slipped out her bedroom window and gone to visit Sabrina. That same week Dana had received her first-ever deficiency reports from school in Spanish and math. The evaluation consisted of an initial session with Dana and her mother, a second session split between individual time with Dana first and then her mother, and a third session that the father attended. The therapist divided this third session between individual time for the father and conjoint time for all three of them.

The genogram produced several interesting facts that documented an increase in the family's stress level. Three months before the clinic visit, the company for which Dana's father was chief corporation counsel had been faced with the real possibility of a hostile takeover. In the same period Dana's maternal grandmother, to whom she was particularly close, found out that she had uterine cancer.

During the evaluation sessions, the therapist, a woman about Mrs. W.'s age, observed Dana scoping her out as if to see whether her attitudes were more similar to Dana's mother or to those of Sabrina's "cool" mother. Dana's mother, on the other hand, seemed mainly interested in whether the therapist believed in law and order, and whether she ever recommended "tough love" groups. Dana's father, distracted by problems in his practice and annoyed at being pulled away from pressing circumstances at work, appeared uninterested. He felt that he had done enough for his daughter by letting her know that she was special to him. Surrounded by many anxiety-producing issues, and by a plethora of interlocking triangles, the therapist chose the following treatment plan.

The first step would be to form a relationship with both Dana and her mother, while avoiding taking sides with one or the other of them. The therapist did this by encouraging Dana to vent about her frustration and anger with her mother, her upset over her grandmother's illness, and what kind of mother she thought would better appreciate a daughter like her. Asked what she thought her mother was most afraid of, Dana responded without hesitation, "That I'll have sex with a whole gang of guys in a dumpster behind the mall."

Turning to Mrs. W., the therapist checked out whether that was her biggest fear, and the mother replied, "One of them." The therapist went on to ask about the other fears and to explore what the mother's life as an early adolescent had been like. This led to a discussion about *her* mother, Dana's grandmother, and opened the issue of her mother's illness. During this part of the session, Dana and her mother forgot their animosity for the moment and shared tears of grief. Dana said that she didn't know what she'd do without her grandmother: "I love her so much."

In a separate session with Dana, the therapist encouraged her to take the initiative with her parents by spelling out on paper her ideas about what was a fair set of guidelines for her conduct and comings and goings. The therapist suggested that Dana might consult Sabrina when preparing this document. Similarly, in a separate session with Dana's parents, the therapist coached them to cease and desist from any criticism or putdowns of Sabrina or her mother. Mr. W. was elected to be the administrative parent and to be the prime negotiator with Dana on the issue of her "guidelines." The therapist asked Mrs. W. whether she thought that raising boys or girls was easier and challenged her to develop a relationship with her daughter that emphasized common interests, spending time, and talking about life. Mrs. W. would accomplish this by loosening her ties with her son and by spending more noninstructional, non-shape-up time with Dana. The therapist asked Mrs. W. to notice how much of her time with Dana was spent giving advice and criticizing versus saying supportive and affectionate things—and then to try to do more of the latter. The idea was to allow her husband to become the "rules parent" and to allow her to evolve into the "fun parent."

The therapy plan tried to deal with some predictable glitches and pitfalls by addressing them early. The therapist asked Mrs. W., for instance, if this experimental plan left her feeling displaced and criticized. Mr. W. was asked how he would make time for this administrative function with everything else he had to do. Dana was told that if she was conflicted and unable to reach her father for clarification, she could call the therapist as a stopgap measure. As Mrs. W. spent less time problem solving for her daughter, she eased up and began to enjoy Dana as a person. This allowed her to spend more time thinking about herself and her own life, what her career would be when Dana left the nest, and what life would be like should her mother die. All these feelings of loss, sadness, confusion, and emptiness, which her preoccupation with Dana had covered up, were encouraged and paid attention to by the therapist. As Mrs. W. moved away emotionally from Dana, she moved into herself, into her loneliness in her marriage and the anxiety of her mother's illness.

Now it was time for the therapist to turn to the peer group triangle consisting of Dana, her friend Sabrina, and Dana's parents. This triangle had Dana in an overly close position with Sabrina, and the over closeness was largely reactive to her parents, who were in the outside position. The triangle was dealt with in two ways. First, the therapist pushed Dana *toward* Sabrina, rather than trying to break them up (which was what the parents were trying, and it would not work in therapy). Second, the therapist tried to get the parents out of the "bad company" position by stopping their criticism of Sabrina. The real issue here wasn't Sabrina's bad influence on Dana, which was not happening at all. The real issue was the intrafamilial stresses and conflicts (like Grandma's illness and Dad's distance), which the family was avoiding by the focus on Sabrina. These issues were tied up in the primary parental triangle to which the therapist could then turn.

This is an example of a peer network triangle in which the parents' fears about bad influence were largely unfounded. Dana had been using Sabrina as a counterpoint to her parents' ideas about what a 13-year-old should be like. However, Sabrina was not in fact a threat to Dana's health or well-being. The main work with the parents was to get them to refrain from a power struggle with Dana about her friend.

It does sometimes happen, however, that a peer triangle can involve real risk or danger. If, for instance, a 13-year-old adolescent's friend is known to use or sell drugs, or to do other truly dangerous things (drag race, carry a gun to school, break into homes), the dan-

ger needs to be dealt with. Palling around with a bad friend is different from palling around with a good one.

However, a triangle is a triangle. The basic principles still apply:
not engaging in a power struggle, and keeping emotional reactivity in
the family as low as possible while keeping thinking as prominent as
possible. If the therapist doesn't emphasize those principles, and the
parents don't or can't put them into practice in the session and at
home, the reactivity will escalate and conservative interventions will
fail. At the next stage, the therapist may be faced with the necessity of
putting the adolescent into the hospital or having to intervene in
some other drastic way.

Besides working on the triangle dynamics, the therapist in these
kinds of cases would have to spend time with the adolescent, asking
whether she believed her friend did sell drugs, and if so, what drew
her to that kind of person? Therapy would also have to address the
question of whether the adolescent is herself using drugs. This can be
handled, if the adolescent denies using and the parents suspect it, by
suggesting to the adolescent (in session alone) that she volunteer for
drug tests as a way of getting this "bogus issue" off the table. The
therapist must deal with the parents about whether they need to take
a position that this friendship is not a good idea and that the adolescent may not contact her friend anymore. If the parents can do this
based on the facts rather than emotional reactivity, they have dealt
functionally with the peer network triangle. Now they should deal
with the fallout from their position in the primary parental triangle
(where the real issue is anyway). The point for the therapist is always
to keep one's eyes on the triangle that is operating, detriangle it, and
move on.

SYMPTOMATIC CHILD TRIANGLES

The success of structural approaches such as Fogarty's, Minuchin's,
and Haley's in producing symptom relief in child-centered families has
been considerable. In recent years, however, these therapeutic maneuvers, in less artistic hands, have at times been used in mechanical and
uncreative ways. For example, the most common structural presentation of a child-centered triangle has the mother and child enmeshed
with the father in the outside, distant, and underfunctioning position.
Fogarty adopted the approach of having the mother *back away* from
the symptomatic child and moving the underinvolved father *in toward*

the child. Fogarty's choice of this intervention was based on his focus on the direction of relationship movement in triangles. It has been his premise for a long time that altering the direction of the movement in a triangle or a marital dyad is the best way to unlock the symptom in an individual and bring relationship processes out into the open so that they are observable to the therapist and the family members.

Minuchin's approach to this triangle concentrates on the boundaries between the family and the therapist and on the importance of generational boundaries within the family system. He always took great care to put himself one-down in relationship to the father, speak to the father first, and then get the father's permission to enter the family. Having done that, he would then work to get the parents to reestablish the appropriate generational boundary between them and their children. Haley's method adds to Minuchin's the importance of a strategic focus for the structural alteration. That is why he had the father introduce a puppy to organize the father–son relationship in the case of the boy with the dog phobia. Each of these methods, when applied in an overly mechanistic way, can lead to an oversimplification of the complex emotional process involved in any dysfunctional family and to a predictable recycling of the symptoms 6 to 8 months after the end of therapy.

The shifts in the direction of relationship movement and structural alteration of the triangles will produce symptom relief, *and* they will uncover underground relationship conflict and emotional states in individuals in the system. Once these conflicts and emotional states are visible, clinical investigation and intervention become much easier. For instance, it wouldn't be unusual to see a dramatic result (as in the case of the dog phobia), only to have the mother, emotionally upset by loss of her intense attachment to her son, become critical of her husband and the therapy and take the puppy back to the store. Although this would be upsetting to the boy and the therapist, we can see such a result as the result of an experimental intervention that tells us something important about the system and the people in it. The results of the experiment have shifted the focus away from the boy and onto the mother's unhappiness and a conflict between the parents. Therefore, we understand symptom relief in a child-centered family as *stage one* in a more comprehensive approach to the multigenerational family process that produced the symptom.

We say this with the full realization that many families will opt for symptomatic relief and nothing more. This "stage one" approach doesn't guarantee that we can alleviate the symptoms in a child by concentrated work on the central mother–father–child triangle without significant fallout elsewhere in the system. However, we can improve the reliability and durability of such results by remaining sensitive to symptom shifts to other family members or relationships and by dealing with them clinically as a natural succession of interrelated processes. Our work in this direction involves the development of a multigenerational paradigm that provides a broad context for viewing the child's symptoms while remaining relevant to the presenting problem.

This clinical paradigm, developed by Guerin and Gordon[4] for dealing with child-centered families, consists of the following set of theoretical assumptions:

1. A child is born into a family with certain constitutional assets and limitations. Among the limitations is a propensity for the type and severity of physical and emotional symptoms he or she may develop during a lifetime. At birth, Mona L. was the fourth child with three older sisters. Her mother dearly wanted to have a son and this, combined with Mona's temperament—a tendency to be cold, to pull back when her mother cuddled her—played into a less close relationship between mother and daughter than Mrs. L. was used to. Mr. L., sensing this distance and believing that Mona had the looks and coloration of his side of the family, felt especially close to Mona.

2. Whether and to what degree these vulnerabilities will emerge over time depend on (a) the basic functioning level of the family system around the time child is born, (b) how well the child's temperament fits the family and his or her sibling position within it, and (c) the amount of internal and external stress the family must absorb and dissipate over its life cycle. Mrs. L. tried especially hard to overcome the cold feeling between her and Mona, and Mr. L. coddled her, so Mona did well in her sibling position. Being the youngest fit naturally into the family system. This arrangement worked well during Mona's early years and into her adolescence.

3. Symptoms will develop when the amount of unbound, or free-floating, anxiety in the family has reached a critical level, that is, beyond the relationship system's ability to bind, diffuse, or dissipate it. As Mona L. was getting on toward 16, her parents were starting to feel the empty-nest syndrome. Most of their children had already gone. Simultaneously, Mrs. L. was undergoing what she called a

---

[4] Guerin and Gordon (1984).

midlife crisis, wondering what she would do when her mothering days were over. Mr. L., a middle manager in a large food brokerage, was laid off and went into a depression.

4. The driving force for this anxiety level will be the development of cluster stress. This is the coming together of a series of transition times and other family events in a quantity sufficient to shake the emotional equilibrium of the family. A classic example of this is the family that is all at once going through the turmoil of adolescence, midlife crises, and grandparental aging and death. In the L. family, Mrs. L.'s focus on her own life and Mr. L.'s distraction by his depression tore the attention of both parents away from Mona. For the first time in her life, Mona felt on her own, independent but isolated within the family.

5. A vulnerable member of the family will absorb the excess anxiety, thereby developing a symptom. Mona L. was vulnerable because of the shift in her longstanding position in the family and began to show the family's anxiety by acting out, openly angry with her mother and feeling responsible for her father's depression.

6. The vulnerable individual most likely to absorb and act out the family's anxiety is the most isolated, invalidated family member, with the least functional leverage in the system. Mona L. had no siblings as allies. Her traditional leverage from her father's attention and her mother's guilt was gone.

7. The symptom serves the function of binding the excess anxiety in the system, allowing the family to maintain its organization or reorganize and continue functioning. As Mona L. developed her symptoms, her father and mother became alarmed at her behavior. They could get off their own problems temporarily and pull together to seek help for Mona. It was only in family therapy for Mona's problem that all the information above came to the surface.

In a symptomatic child triangle, one parent is overly close to and overinvolved with one or more of the children, and the other parent is in the distant and critical position. A wife who is an emotional pursuer, frustrated with her husband's distance, turns to pursuing her children. One child, sensitive to the mother's upset, gets caught in the triangle and begins to act out in some way. The child's acting out brings the parents together as they avoid their personal conflicts to cooperate in worrying about the child. So the marital conflict is covered over.

Karl H. was an 11-year-old only child, whose parents had been treated for marital conflict 3 years before their presentation with

Karl. In calling for an appointment, Mrs. H. was quick to tell the therapist that "everything is fine" between her and her husband; the problem was that Karl has started to do poorly in school and to act "very fresh" at home. In addition, there had been several episodes of lying and stealing. The genogram and history revealed several losses to Karl several months before the onset of his symptoms. His parents blamed these losses for Karl's behavior (although Mr. H. thought that his wife's laxity with Karl also had something to do with his behavior). Both parents were involved with Karl, but Mrs. H. was clearly overly close. Mr. H., whose work demanded very long hours, yielded to her in spite of his occasional disapproval.

Karl's best friend had moved to another city, and Karl really missed him. They did speak on the phone, however, and occasionally saw each other when the friend was visiting his grandparents. The second loss involved Karl's maternal grandmother, whose (apparently successful) bout with cancer had left her unable to see Karl as much as had been her custom. Mrs. H. acknowledged that she herself had been extremely upset by her mother's cancer, but she expressed confidence that her mother was now fine. The third, and probably most severe loss to Karl, involved his paternal grandmother, who had lived with them and cared for Karl all his life. About the same time Karl's maternal grandmother got cancer and his friend moved away, his mother and paternal grandmother had a dispute that ended in Mrs. H. asking her mother-in-law to leave. She did and went to live with a daughter.

Mr. H. had no great fondness for his mother, but he had given his father, to whom he was very attached, an oath on his father's deathbed that he would care for her. He denied being angry with his wife for the way things turned out but anticipated that his mother would one day return. When he said this in session, his wife visibly flinched.

Many triangles appear from this case narrative: Mr. H., and his mother, and father; Mr. H. and Mrs. H., and Mr. H.'s mother; Karl, Mrs. H., and Karl's grandmothers (two different triangles); and Karl and his parents. These all interlocked with one another, and the emotional energy from each of them fed the process in all the others. For a complete cure of this case, all should have been addressed, but this family didn't stay in treatment long enough to do so. The therapist did provide symptom relief by first addressing Karl and his parents, since that is the triangle most likely making Karl feel caught.

The first step was to suggest that Mr. H. take charge of Karl's behavior, leaving it to Mr. H. to lay down the rules and deal with any violations. This revealed Mrs. H.'s depression and her anxiety about her own mother. At this point, the therapist evaluated Mrs. H. and began appropriate treatment for depression. Talking with Mrs. H. about her mother led to talking about Mr. H.'s mother and what it was like to live with her all Mrs. H.'s married life. With Karl absent from the sessions, the therapist at this juncture, began to deal with the underground issue about Mr. H.'s mother. At this point the family stopped treatment.

However, Karl and his parents got some relief, even if temporary, from Karl's symptoms. That's what the family wanted, and they left when they got it. Karl's symptoms will recur in one form or another, however, because the underlying triangles are untouched. Since the family got some symptom relief, presumably they will return, and the therapist will have another chance.

In this chapter, we have presented the three major ways in which child and adolescent triangles present clinically. The following chapter elaborates more fully on the intrafamilial, symptomatic, child and adolescent triangles seen more frequently in clinical practice.

CHAPTER TWELVE

Symptomatic Child and Adolescent Triangles within the Family

Intrafamilial child and adolescent triangles may be subdivided into five categories: the target child, the parent and sibling triangle, the sibling subsystem triangle, the three-generational triangle, and stepfamily triangles. Each of these will be considered in turn.

THE TARGET CHILD

A child who is special to one parent may become the target of resentment by the other parent who is the outsider in the triangle. This parent's anger may be directed at the target child for several reasons. Among them may be the child's possession of qualities that resemble those of the other parent, his or her resemblance to the spouse's extended family, or just the child's specialness to the other spouse. The parent who is targeting the child for anger and criticism is displacing that anger and criticism from someone else in the system, usually his or her spouse.

Target children often have internalized versions of both parents, which wage war inside them. People experience this war as a tension, and target children feel caught between their parents. They cannot tolerate their parents' conflict because of the upset it triggers inside them. As a result, they behave in self-destructive ways because of their own emotional upset, and parents join in an artificial unity concerning a troublesome child. Instead of a man and woman who have conflicts with each other, they become parents united in their concern for the child.

Structurally, these target child triangles usually present as an overly close relationship between symptomatic child and mother, with the father in the outside position, distant from both his wife and child. At least two standard intervention techniques are available in this clinical situation. The first intervention attempts to bridge the distance between a father and a symptomatic child. It does this by organizing their relationship around an activity or object of mutual interest. Father and son might be encouraged to spend time together doing something both find interesting and pleasant: perhaps watching a sporting event together; or having the father coach his son's little league team; or just sitting in the family room watching television. The important thing is that, while doing these things, father and son not get into any discussion of problems but just learn to be comfortable with each other. They should also be advised to make an effort to avoid discussing the mother.

The other technique prescribes a *bilateral* intervention of moving the father in to take responsibility for all of the parenting functions for the symptomatic child. Simultaneously, it instructs the overinvolved mother to retire temporarily from her mothering role: that is, to distance from the symptomatic child and to refrain from instructing her husband or making editorial comments about his relationship with the child.

Both methods can be effective in quickly relieving the child's symptoms and opening access to other dysfunctional processes in the family that are fueling those symptoms. However, the therapist must remain aware of some limitations of these methods. First, the symptomatic child is often highly sensitized to the level of emotional upset in the mother. The structural rearrangements that these methods prescribe will predictably raise the mother's level of anxiety and internal upset, probably increasing the child's anxiety. The father's increasing involvement with his son or daughter may insulate the child from this upset. However, the mother's anxiety may override the insulating effect of the father's increased involvement. This happens if the father has significant difficulty carrying out his portion of the task or if the mother's anxiety gets raised beyond a critical level. (If the symptomatic child happens to be an adolescent girl, the above prescription is developmentally inappropriate, for it is essential at this time that children establish an effective relationship bridge with the same-sex parent.)

When the mother's anxiety threatens to reach a critical level, the problem can be dealt with effectively by working with the mother, either alone or in the family sessions, to develop an awareness of how the symptomatic child is sensitized to increased anxiety in her. This can often be effected simply by asking a few process questions, such as, "Have you ever noticed which of the children seems most affected by your upsets even when you're trying hard to keep the upset to yourself?" "Which of the children seems sensitized in that way to your husband?" The therapist addresses the same questions to the father. We can then ask the symptomatic child a series of questions: "Can you tell when your mom is upset?" "How?" "What does it do to your insides?" "How do you behave when you're feeling like that?" If these questions are successful, the emotional process that is feeding the anxiety in the family will be opened up and dealt with and the anxiety decreased. This usually relieves the symptoms in the child and defines the sources of anxiety and the conflictual emotional process elsewhere in the family so we can deal with them, too, more functionally.

The father's criticism and negativity in reaction to the child's specialness to the mother, with the father feeling the discomfort of the outside position, is significant. It focuses the therapy process onto how much the symptomatic child's close relationship with or behavioral similarity to the other parent is triggering the attacking parent into criticism and negativity.

It must be kept in mind that whatever intervention is chosen must be contextually relevant to the family. The more closed the system, the more intense the projection process toward the child. The more concrete and the less cognitively oriented the family is, the more the situation calls for a simple structural maneuver.

Gloria and Bruce V. came to the therapist for an evaluation. The presenting problem was their 6-year-old son Justin, who was having tantrums at home and at school. He also had encopresis. When asked to do almost anything at home, he would rage, swear at his parents and at his mother in particular. At school he would wander around the class, bother the other students, demand constant attention from the teacher, and often refuse to obey. To the therapist, this sounded initially like hyperactivity and therapy started by having the parents agree on their approach to Justin. They would expose him gradually to discipline in a consistent way, with rewards for good behavior and consequences when he didn't obey.

This behavior modification initially produced some good results. Still, there were apparently differences between Gloria and Bruce about how each really believed their son should be handled. They began to argue about the correct way to handle Justin. A power struggle was going on between them about the boy. Gloria wanted to be more understanding of Justin, and Bruce wanted to be stricter, with fewer discussions. Gloria explained more often, and Bruce threw his hands up and withdrew. Thus, they neutralized each other.

Dealing with this conflict between the parents finally elicited the comment from Gloria that Bruce was treating Justin the same way he treated her—abruptly, without patience or understanding. As the anxiety in the family shifted toward what was going on with Gloria and Bruce and away from Justin, Justin's behavior improved. It *could* improve because it was no longer serving to bind the anxiety between and inside Gloria and Bruce. Therapy then went on to focus on Gloria, Bruce, their emotional states, and their relationship.

It should be said that most target child triangles are much more entrenched in some families than in others. It's often not so easy to reach the marital discord that underlies this type of triangle. Because the marital relationship in a child-centered family is the most sensitive one, it is the most protected one. Unless we keep in mind that there is a triangle present, we may fall for the protective moves by the parents to focus on the symptomatic child.

By the same token, it's a mistake to move the therapy process into the marital relationship too fast. The family will probably disappear from therapy. We have to be patient and let the process evolve. We should stay alert and watch for openings—such as depression in a mother when she pulls back from over closeness with her child or a father's reluctance to move in and develop a relationship with his child.

Awareness of triangles and the detriangling process is clarifying and productive of change in just about every family situation. The results can often lead to seemingly magical improvement in the symptomatic child and, of course, the eruption of a submerged marital problem.

THE PARENT AND SIBLING TRIANGLE

Besides the two forms of primary parental triangle discussed above, there are several interlocking, auxiliary triangles that we must define in order fully to understand the process in a child-centered family and give ourselves as many therapeutic options as possible. The first of these triangles is the sibling–parent triangle, involving the symptomatic child, a sibling, and one parent. This triangle is potentially present in any family constellation with at least two children, but it is perhaps most often seen in the single-parent family.

In most single-parent households headed by a mother, the mother needs to leave home base every day to go to work. This fact creates a leadership vacuum at home. Usually the oldest daughter fills the vacuum, taking over as head of the household while the mother is away at work. Putting the oldest in the position can also happen, of course, in dual-career, two-parent households, but it is usually less dramatic. The oldest daughter often ends up in a difficult position. She assumes considerable responsibility without any real power and then must vacate her position of authority and go back to being just one of the kids when her mother returns.

When we combine this pattern with the possibility of the oldest daughters' "specialness" to her absent father, a great deal of potential conflict springs up between the mother and her oldest daughter. This conflict most often takes the form of increasing criticism of the oldest daughter by the mother, which is a double standard of conduct for the oldest daughter and younger siblings. The oldest daughter keeps her distance when her mother is around. She expresses her negativity in passive–aggressive ways toward the mother and in openly punitive ways toward her youngest sister, the mother's special child. The parentified child sometimes gets into dangerous behavior outside the house and sometimes makes suicide gestures.

These families often present with the symptoms in the youngest, and if family intervention takes the form of increasing the mother's focus on the youngest, her symptoms will get worse. The worsening of symptoms is the result of increasing pressure from the oldest daughter to youngest daughter in response to the mother's attention. If, on the other hand, we focus the intervention on exposing and decreasing the conflict between a mother and oldest daughter, we remove the sibling pressure from the youngest and her symptoms will disappear.

Janis L., a single-parent mother of three girls, sought help for her family with a behavior problem with Ginny, her youngest. Careful watching of the process in this family revealed the fact that Janis had a special, overly close relationship with Ginny. She worried about her a great deal and spent an inordinate amount of relationship time with her. Ginny was fiercely loyal to her mother and withheld herself emotionally from her nonresident father, Jack. Amy, the oldest sister, was a physical and behavioral "clone" of her father. She also resented her baby sister. Sue, the middle daughter, appeared to operate in all of the different factions in the family well and floated free of the overt and covert conflicts.

Here, the therapist worked on two interlocking triangles. The most active, proximate one involved Janis, her oldest child, Amy, and the symptomatic youngest, Ginny. The therapist surfaced and placed the covert conflict between Janis and Amy in the context of the triangle made up of Janis, Ginny, and her absent father. As Janis and Amy dealt with the conflict between them, the pressure between Amy and Ginny diminished, and Ginny became symptom-free. Over the long haul, this also opened the possibility for Ginny to have a more involved relationship with her father.

The most instructive part of this case is the demonstration of a key relationship triangle underlying the presenting symptoms in the youngest child. If the therapist had not discovered this triangle through clinical experimentation, its neglect would have prolonged the negative therapeutic result. Picking up the oldest daughter's difficult position in the family and her indirect involvement in her sister's symptoms allowed the therapist to formulate a successful plan of intervention.

THE SIBLING SUBSYSTEM TRIANGLE

The second auxiliary triangle of clinical importance is the sibling subsystem triangle. Because an adult, usually a parent, commonly initiates therapy, it's easy to formulate the troubled system to include the parents. We expect them as adults to be in control of the family. Children are young and don't have it together yet. We expect squabbling between siblings in families, and we often perceive their struggles as misbehavior concretized as who-did-what-to-whom and who-started-it. Often parents blame one child for sibling fights while they let the others off. Thus, we may overlook interlocking triangles among the siblings. For example, two siblings who are for their mother and against their father in a divorce dispute may put pressure on another sibling to separate from Dad and sign on with Mom. Or, one child in the family may get his or her identity not by trying to become someone, but by isolating from his or her siblings and trying to be reactively different from them. The triangle that first leaps out when we see a family, may not be the only significant triangle in the family.

The sibling subsystem deserves investigation in any child-centered family. First, its cohesion–fragmentation index needs examination. This index represents the degree to which the siblings are emotionally connected or distant from one another. A simple and productive way of learning this is to ask the children how often they band together behind closed doors to complain about their parents. Families with a well-functioning, cohesive sibling subsystem will enthusiastically endorse that activity, while those that are fragmented will respond as if the therapist is speaking a foreign language.

Our experience has been that fragmented sibling subsystems are most frequently present in families with anorexia, severe behavior disorders, and psychotic-level process. The symptom-bearing child is invariably the one in the outside position in the triangles that exist among the siblings. In these clinical situations, parents will often strongly resist the inclusion of the better-functioning, symptom-free children in therapy sessions. When this happens, the therapist says that the other children must participate. She or he may temporarily isolate the sibling subsystem by working with the siblings alone in some sessions. The therapist does this in an attempt to increase their connection with each other and alter the dysfunctional sibling triangles.

The S. family came to therapy 3 months after their oldest, a son, Andrew, left for college. Their middle daughter, Katie, a sophomore in high school, was showing symptoms of progressive anorexia. She was complaining of being fat, though her weight was below normal for her height. She was dieting and was spending 2 or 3 hours a day working out on the Stairmaster at the exercise salon she belonged to. One other child, Hillary, age 13, was an eighth-grader at a local parochial school. Mr. S. was a successful businessman, and Mrs. S. was a part-time foreign language tutor at the local high school. Andrew had been a superstar in high school, lettering in football, baseball, and basketball. He had been a straight-A student, a volunteer at the community hospital, and beloved in the community. He had a special relationship with both of his parents and his baby sister, Hillary. His relationship with his symptomatic sister, Katie, had always been cordial, but Andrew often thought that her whiny behavior, moodiness, and clinging were uncalled for. Katie was born 3 days after the death of her maternal grandfather, and since early childhood had been the barometer of family upsets, especially the mother's. Although she had always admired her big brother, she resented his closeness to Hillary and felt on the outside. In family therapy both parents resisted the involvement of the two asymptomatic children, especially bringing Andrew home from college on weekends for special family sessions. The therapist insisted, and Andrew's involvement proved crucial on two fronts: First, it allowed the family's intense reactivity to his departure for college to surface, and second, it established the basis for increased communication and relationship contact between Andrew and Katie. The latter had a positive effect on Katie's symptoms.

Structure

In this sibling-subsystem triangle, Katie occupied the outsider position. Even when this triangle was dormant, its form remained fixed. Sometimes Katie and her younger sister would move closer around "girl issues," but in Katie's mind the shadow of her "special" older brother always made its presence felt in the sisters' relationship.

Process

The developmental history that preceded symptom formation in Katie significantly influenced the structure and process in this triangle. Another factor was the intrusion of system-wide anxiety and emotional arousal surrounding Andrew's departure for college. When Katie was born, Andrew was already firmly entrenched in the "favorite child" slot. The fact that he was the first grandchild in a family that overvalued male children was a major contributor to this phenomenon. In addition, it was likely that Katie's birth, occurring so close to her maternal grandfather's death, especially sensitized her to her mother's anxiety and emotional distress. Since we could assume that the mother's emotional distress was significant in the early months and years of Katie's life, we could attribute some of Katie's early life problems with adjustments to feeding and sleeping schedules to that. These early life problems also attracted a significant amount of attention from her mother, which didn't endear her to her younger sister. She was used to being the sole object of concern and attention. In addition, Katie's way of responding to internal tension was to somatize, withdraw socially, and become generally passive and whiny. These behaviors formed a temperamental profile that didn't fit with the expectation of her family any more than they pleased her older brother.

At the age of 2, her parents had confronted Katie with the arrival of her baby sister, Hillary, and the old process repeated itself. Hillary was born with a sunny disposition, which fit perfectly with her sibling position as what we call a "free-floating youngest." In times of increased tension, Hillary responded in two ways. She became a comforter and cheerer-upper of family members, or as she got older, she would increase the pace of her social schedule.

When Andrew left for college, his father shifted what little relationship time he had to his younger daughter. These events left the mother bereft over the developmental inevitability of her son's departure, and Katie sensitized to her mother's emotional distress. Katie was not tied in a functional way in any other relationship. The family emotional process had its way, and Katie's somatizing tendencies led to the development of the symptoms of an eating disorder.

Function

Katie was the child most adversely affected by an increase in tension in her mother. Her outsider position in the sibling subsystem triangle didn't afford her any sibling support in times of tension, or for that matter most of the time. The family didn't deal well with upset in the mother, or any expression of negative affect by her. This sibling subsystem triangle afforded the family a way of not focusing on the mother's upset and a way of displacing its incompetence at dealing with the expression of negative emotion by making both of them Katie's problem.

Intervention

On the level of the sibling subsystem triangle, therapy needed to work to improve the attachment between the two sisters. The therapist did this by challenging the younger sister with the fact that female-to-female relationships in this family weren't satisfactory and by opening the issue of emotional reaction to brother Andrew's departure. Bringing Andrew home for a weekend session provided the opportunity to deal with the long-term issue of Andrew's emotional reaction to Katie's "illnesses."

In addition, the therapy needed to explore Katie's position in the interlocking primary parental triangle and to address the father's less than adequate support of the mother and his weak attachment to Katie. It was important in working with the sibling subsystem triangle to make it explicit that the siblings weren't responsible for each other's well being and physical or mental health. They were only responsible for fostering a functional attachment to each other, with an awareness of the potentially destructive nature of fixed triangles.

THE THREE-GENERATIONAL TRIANGLE

The third type of clinically important *auxiliary triangle* in child-centered families is the three-generational triangle consisting of the symptomatic child, a parent, and a grandparent. The process in a three-generational triangle may be set in motion at birth, or even before. There are two major pathways by which this can occur.

The first pathway for setting in motion the three-generational triangle concerns what we may call the battle of the grandmothers. In the time just before and immediately following the baby's birth, the family system may go through a series of relationship maneuvers. These are attempts to establish the primacy of bonding between the new infant and one side of the extended family. The least subtle aspects of this process play out in the viewing room of the hospital nursery, when anxious relatives cast their votes for the family member or side of the family the baby most resembles. (The mother's mother: "She's so beautiful; she looks just like my mother!" The father's mother: "Do you think? I think she looks just like her father.") The geographic proximity of a more cohesive family makes this process more immediate and observable. In more disengaged or (geographically) scattered families, the process may be more remote. A parent can develop an unconscious reactivity to a child's resemblance to an important but distant family member.

The emotional process triggered by the death, most often of a grandparent, but sometimes of another important member of the extended family, creates a second major pathway through which a child may get caught in a three-generational triangle. People put the anxiety and upset surrounding that loss into the relationship between a parent and the particular child born in the period of about 2 years before or after the grandparent's death. This child is sensitized to anxiety in a particular parent or to an increase in family emotional arousal following upon an event like a grandparent's death. From being sensitized, the child is vulnerable, at least through childhood and adolescence, to future increases in that parent's anxiety or in the family's level of emotional arousal, and he or she may act out in a variety of ways.

When his mother was pregnant with Mitch B., her father had a heart attack at age 52. He had a second, fatal, attack 2 months after Mitch was born. Mrs. B. had been very close to her father, and his first heart attack had frightened her badly. When he died, she had gone into a clinical depression. When Mitch was 13, his mother's mother was diagnosed with cancer. Within weeks of her mother's diagnosis, Mrs. B. was getting phone calls from Mitch's middle school that Mitch was cutting classes. His behavior escalated into violating no-smoking rules in the school building, getting into fistfights, and screaming at teachers. Mrs. B. brought him to treatment, where the therapist's hypothesis was that Mitch was responding to his mother's upset about her mother's illness and that Mitch's response could be traced back to Mrs. B.'s father's illness and death around the time of Mitch's birth. The therapist opened discussions with Mitch and Mrs. B. about her parents and the sadness she felt about their loss.

Even during her pregnancy, a mother's upset when a significant member of the extended family, particularly a grandparent, dies may sensitize the child to increased anxiety and emotional upheaval in later years on that side of the extended family. The mechanism for the transmission of this anxiety is simplest to track when it is a death in the mother's family: We can postulate the mother's emotional response and its impact on the developing fetus as the mechanism behind the sensitization of that child to upset on that side of the extended family.

When the child's sensitization is to the father's side of the family, two factors may be important. One is the extensive involvement of the paternal grandmother in the early years of the child's life. Later developments in the grandmother's life, such as the death of her husband, will greatly affect that particular child. The other factor is the situation in which the child's mother is cut off from her extended family and has adopted her husband's family as her own. Here a traumatic event or increased anxiety in the husband's family has a profound crossover effect on her and thence on the child who is sensitized to her. This effect is compounded when the mother, believing she is an "adopted" daughter in her husband's family, is surprised to find herself in the outsider position at the time of upset.

The J. family came to therapy with Brenda, a 14-year-old high school freshman referred by the school for antisocial behavior. The assistant principal had repeatedly caught her smoking in the lavatory and cutting classes. The last straw for the school was a fistfight Brenda got into with another girl about a loan the other girl hadn't repaid. Her father and his second wife brought Brenda for the first session. Brenda lived with her mother, but her mother thought therapy was a waste of time. She had had 8 years of individual therapy following her divorce and was now practicing transcendental meditation with her latest lover. To her, Brenda's behavior was normal for her age and "She would grow out of it." Mr. J., with his second wife in agreement, framed the problem as inadequate mothering. Brenda defended her mother and said that although she was "flaky," she had not been the one to leave. Her father had, when Brenda was 3.

Brenda asked to see the therapist alone. He agreed, and when they met, she told him that she had heard from a friend that the therapist understood kids better than most adults. So she wanted to tell him how it really was. She told him her understanding of how her father and mother had married when they were both very young. She had the misfortune of having been born when neither of them knew what they really wanted. From Brenda's perspective, both her parents had found themselves new lives, and she didn't fit into either one of them. The therapist asked her who besides her parents had been a special adult to her. Brenda became tearful immediately and softly said, "My grandmother." She looked utterly miserable and alone. The therapist remembered from the genogram that the paternal grandmother had died 6 months earlier. He asked about her and her death. With tears streaming down her face, Brenda told him that she could always count on her grandmother being there—now it seemed "like there was no one."

The therapist asked Brenda if she had talked to her father or her mother's mother about her grief. She said no but agreed to meet in separate sessions with each of them to talk about her grandmother's death and where she saw herself in its aftermath. They held both of those sessions. After listening to Brenda Mr. J. revealed his own unresolved grief for his mother. He also felt some of his guilt about his mother and Brenda and about his long-term distance from both of them. The maternal grandmother confessed her respect for her departed counterpart and her jealousy of Brenda's special relationship with her.

A week after that session, Brenda called the therapist to say she felt much better. She said that, since both her grandmother and mother were against coming back, she thought it wasn't worth the hassle. She promised to call if things got bad again.

Mr. J. came in for another visit to report on the school's positive reaction to Brenda's improvement and his willingness to continue therapy if the therapist thought it necessary. The therapist told him just to keep in touch and let him know how things were going. They could always come back if the problem reappeared. Six months later the father called to say things were continuing to go well. He was spending more relationship time with his daughter. They had been to the cemetery to visit his mother's grave. The maternal grandmother and Brenda were doing very well, and Brenda's mother was still meditating.

One final note. Triangles with the children can take these or many other forms, and the therapist must treat them carefully. When marital conflict isn't the presenting problem, therapists should avoid the temptation to make it explicit prematurely.

STEPFAMILY TRIANGLES

A last variant of intrafamilial triangles are those that occur in stepfamilies. A very common story is that of Alan and Elizabeth H., both previously divorced and in their middle 40s. Both carried emotional scars from their divorces, and each had given up hope that there was a chance in life for them to recapture love in another relationship. Because of their pain, their courtship had been prolonged over 4 or 5 years. During this time, they gradually grew more intimate and would sometimes sleep over at one or the other's house when the children were not around. Five years after meeting, they decided that time had assuaged their hurt and that marriage was possible.

They were married very soon after making the decision, and the marriage united Alan, Elizabeth, Elizabeth's two teenage daughters, and Alan's son and daughter when they visited him. All went well until Alan tried to enforce housekeeping rules on Elizabeth's 16-year-old daughter, Jane. Jane became sullen and told Alan, "You're not my father." She then went to Elizabeth and complained about Alan, telling Elizabeth that he was "just like my father was." Over time, after many complaints from Jane and many defenses from Alan, Elizabeth began to think she had made the same mistake in her second marriage as in her first—choosing an abusive mate.

Once started, this triangular process only got worse over the next 2 years. Finally Elizabeth suggested therapy, and Alan agreed.

As in all the other triangles we've mentioned in our discussion of marital conflict, stepfamily triangles allow for the avoidance of issues between husband and wife. Often entwined in the marital issues are pieces of unfinished business from each spouse's previous marriage. At the heart of triangulation are questions of loyalties in relationships. The biological tie to children and the historical and financial tie to previous spouses present many opportunities for the stepfamily marriage to fall into conflict. ("You're not my father. I don't have to listen to you." Or, "I know she's your daughter and not mine, but you shouldn't let her stay out this late.") Often the honeymoon is over before the wedding takes place, as the family systems involved begin reverberating in response to the impending marriage. Added to this already complicated picture is the potential of four sets of (ex-) in-laws and worried grandparents who fear that a remarriage will disrupt their relationships with grandchildren.

Types of Stepfamily Triangles

Clinically, remarried couples often present with one or more of the following triangles evident.

The Wicked Stepparent Triangle

In this triangle, open warfare breaks out between stepchildren and stepparent, with the spouse who is the natural parent pulled back and forth between a child and new spouse. The stepparent is usually critical of the stepchild, and the stepchild, often an adolescent, is enraged at this interloper's behavior toward her or him: "Who does he think he is?" The biological parent often feels torn apart by the need to defend one or both parties in the conflict. It seems like a no-win situation.

The Perfect Stepparent Triangle

The stepparent is often operating off an implicit demand from the spouse that he or she take over the stepchild as his or her own. In this triangle, the stepparent operates as the rescuer, moving toward the stepchild to "fix" the child, or perhaps to make up to the child for the past. The biological parent is in a distant, more comfortable position, initially delighted with the closeness between a child and the new spouse. Trouble arises when the stepparent inevitably fails as a parent over time, and the biological parent becomes increasingly critical. The stepchild also becomes reactive as the stepparent attempts to fill the distance between the biological parent and the child. We most commonly see this turn of events with an overly close stepmother and a distant biological father, or with a stepfather trying to make it up to a stepchild for a biological father absent because of death or divorce.

Cheryl and William C. illustrate the problem in the perfect stepparent triangle. They came to therapy because Cheryl's 7-year-old daughter, Bo, was acting willful and was impossible for Cheryl to handle. Cheryl, 26, had never been married to Sal, Bo's father. She and William, 28, had been married for 2 years. Bo called William Daddy, and she called Sal, whom she saw once a week, Dad. William did most of the talking at the evaluation, explaining that Sal was a beer-drinking, generally immature man whose behavior confused Bo. He said that he and Cheryl had tried to warn Bo about Sal's behavior, but they felt that continuing to see him was important for Bo. Cheryl admitted that she could not deal with Sal and that she relied heavily on William to do this for her. She also had difficulty dealing with Bo, who apparently ran her mother ragged. Teaching Cheryl how to deal both with her daughter and with her daughter's father was essential here. Helping William find a way to have a relationship with Bo that was more appropriate for a stepparent was also important.

This situation shows how a stepparent like William may be operationally the father, in the sense that Cheryl expected him to control Bo. However, William had no real title and therefore had responsibility without authority. It was Cheryl who had the title and the authority, but she didn't use it, and she expected William to deal with Sal and Bo for her. The therapeutic move was to persuade Cheryl to go one-on-one with Sal and with Bo, and to help William develop some kind of effective position in relation to Bo. This should help clear up the confusion about who is dealing with whom about what. It should also provide Bo with some structure and make her easier to deal with. If this isn't done, Bo can be expected to continue acting out within the family and then to transfer his behavior outside the family. Eventually the disorganization could become so great that William and Cheryl might even dissolve their marriage.

The Ghost of the Ex-Spouse Triangle

This triangle is characterized by the wife or husband being reactive to the mate's relationship with a former spouse, usually the mother of the stepchildren. Issues of alimony and child support, and the nature and frequency of contact with the ex-wife, can create open conflict between the marital partners. Whether the previous marriage ended through divorce or death, feeling like a priority in the family is often difficult for the new spouse. If the marriage ended through divorce, conflicts over money and children often tie the spouse to the previous mate. If the marriage ended through death, the ghost of the previous spouse can be very present and even idealized.

An example of the latter are Todd and Pam Y. Pam's first husband hanged himself 2 years before she met Todd. After their marriage she and Todd moved into the apartment that had belonged to her first husband and had been left to Pam in his will. Todd was passive and seemingly disinterested in anything to do with their new home. Pam was angry and felt beset with all the responsibility for their daily living. Todd wouldn't even change a light bulb. Tasks that he volunteered for he would forget. Pam was fed up and felt conned, since before they were married Todd had been very active in their life together. In therapy, Todd began to express his feeling that he was an outsider in his home. He could feel Pam's first husband's influence everywhere in the apartment. He also felt that Pam was very controlling and would not allow him to have his own territory. Although Pam's first husband was dead, he lived on between the couple.

A similar process with different content goes on in a remarriage after a divorce. The tone of the triangle can be different depending on whether the divorce was amicable or bitter, but the process is similar. Stu and Shana H. are an example. Shana bristled every time she learned that Stu was going to a school meeting with Peggy, his first wife. It seemed to Shana that he was at Peggy's beck and call and that Peggy was a higher priority than she. Stu had been married to Peggy for 15 years. They had three children, two of whom had learning disabilities. Stu, an educator, believed that he should be involved with Peggy when it came to the children. Shana believed that Peggy used this to undercut Shana's marriage to Stu. When she would confront Stu with this, he accused her of being selfish and difficult to get along with. It became such a problem between them that it brought them to therapy.

In both of these situations, the breakup of a marriage and the death of a spouse (Todd and Pam; Shana and Stu), we need an overview that includes some family members who are "absent." These absent members are nevertheless active participants in family triangles. In cases where one spouse has died, therapists should direct some of their effort to helping the formerly married spouse to structure the divorced relationship so that it doesn't continue to interfere with the second marriage. Otherwise there will be a ghost in the marriage, and this ghost will be a real but unrecognized interference in the marital or parental relationships. This intrusion can lead to all kinds of conflict, over closeness in marital or parental twosomes with someone left out in the cold, or another triangle with its roots in an unrecognized triangle from a previous relationship.

The Grandparent Triangle

This triangle is especially pertinent if the grandparents are forced to deal with a former son- or daughter-in-law with whom they had a good deal of reactivity before the divorce. For example, if a husband sees his mother-in-law as having been too interfering and influential with his wife, he may have a good bit of trouble allowing her a grandmother role after divorce and remarriage. Holding in-laws responsible in part for the marital breakup may also contribute to problems around visitations for grandparents.

Treatment Goals in Stepfamily Triangles

After the therapist identifies the most relevant stepfamily triangle and surfaces the process, clinical management involves *shifting the relationships so that they reflect the real and functional picture of each stepfamily member's role.* For example, stepparents who attempt to act as if they are the biological parents frequently run into difficulty. A stepparent the children see as "good" or "wicked" may be moving too quickly or attempting to cross biological boundaries. He or she needs to carve out a more appropriate role evolved over time with the child. Remarried parents need to have realistic expectations of each other as stepparents. Therapists must make the ghosts of ex-spouses explicit and get the family to deal openly with them. This demands an acceptance of the fact that the bond between former spouses is never broken when the marriage has produced offspring, but lives on for generations to come.

The second goal in dealing with the stepfamily triangle is *to address the interlocking triangles that are influencing the central triangle.* In a remarriage, the first marriage and the new relationship may have pushed relationships between the biological children into the background. The hurts and anger attached to these relationships become displaced onto the stepfamily. A father cut off from his own children may be moving in on his stepchildren to shape them up or make them his. He may be doing this without regard for the loss he has suffered by not having a relationship with his own children. When met with a rebuff from his stepchildren, his reactivity can be intense.

People inevitably expose scar tissue from the previous marriage as they move from their position in the triangle and begin to look at the nature of the fuel for the movement. *Unfinished business, mainly the buried bitter bank from the previous relationship, needs to be explored.* This is the third goal in treating stepfamily triangles.

In triangles that involve children, therapists should try to get parents to go one-on-one with the child and to avoid interfering with each other. As the child improves, conflict between the parents usually unfolds. Parents often see this as a deterioration in the family when, in fact, it represents a stage in the evolution of the family toward function. This leads naturally into the types of triangles therapists see in marriages.

If therapists don't recognize and understand triangles, therapy is apt to be centered around an intrapsychic process in a way that doesn't fully acknowledge the force and power of triangular interpersonal dynamics. Children are likely to define their difficulties in terms of their relationship with one parent or the other and not realize that by focusing on that relationship they are missing the larger picture. For instance, by defending mother and attacking father, they miss the difficulties they have in their relationship with mother because it "looks" so good. By focusing on a "bad" father, they miss the part they play in the problem—the only part they can change. It's crucial to define the problem in terms of triangles, to get people to go one-on-one with each other, and to define their own parts in the problem in terms of this one on one relationship. When therapists use this paradigm, the internal dynamics of the self aren't lost—they manifest themselves more quickly and more clearly.

CHAPTER THIRTEEN

Conclusion: Becoming a "Triangle Doctor"

THE PERVASIVENESS OF TRIANGLES IN RELATIONSHIPS AND IN THERAPY

Normal people and mental health professionals automatically think about ones and twos. When things go badly in our lives or in therapy, each of us quickly moves to questions like, "What did I do wrong?" or "Who did me in?" Our purpose in this book has been to facilitate our readers' ability to think about threes and to recognize triangles when they do occur.

One way of looking at life is to see it as a never-ending series of relationship triangles to be recognized and resolved. From conception on, we are part of our primary parental triangle. As we negotiate childhood, triangles with our siblings, grandparents, aunts, uncles, and cousins dot the relationship landscape. Adolescence, with its famous emotional storms, makes triangles inside and outside the family explicit and easy to see. As young adults move to form their own marital and nuclear family units, relationship triangles multiply in number and in interlocking complexity. If we are aware of the developmental density of triangles in our own lives and in the lives of our patients, we can more easily find, define, and neutralize the specific triangles that may be defeating us at a particular moment in time.

For purposes of efficiency and cost effectiveness, as clinicians we deal with the matter at hand—whether anxiety, depression, or relationship conflict—by freezing it in time, analyzing it, and treating it.

This doesn't take away from the fact that each symptom or clinical episode, with its accompanying triangle, is just one in a connected series that has occurred over time.

Our lives and our therapeutic efforts are complicated immeasurably by the often invisible power of relationship triangles. Remember the time when you were 7 years old, on a neighborhood exploration with your best friend, and you wanted to cut across the frozen pond on the way to the candy store? Your friend said his mother wouldn't let him. Undaunted, you did it anyway, and he ran home and told your big sister. She not only came and got you, and dropped you home before you got a chance to buy your candy, but she also ratted on you to your mother. Your mother sent you to your room with the familiar threat: Wait until your father gets home. It was bad enough that your father thought your big sister was perfect and you left a lot to be desired, even though you could already dribble a basketball at age 7.

Did you ever tell your best friend your deepest, darkest secret only to arrive at school the next day and find a group of the most popular and powerful kids gathered in a corner of the schoolyard laughing together in a way that by instinct told you that your friend had told? Now, for the rest of the year, you'd be an outcast. Or in college, when you found out your friend was pursuing your sweetheart? Then you grew up, went to graduate school, found a life partner, and received an intense postgraduate course in mothers-in-law.

Triangles surrounded you when, in clinical practice, little boys who were targets of their fathers' criticism, husbands who couldn't control their libidinal compulsions, and wives driven to depression by the critical squeeze of their mothers and their husbands kept finding their way to your office. It is just this pervasiveness of triangles and of the fallout they produce that inspired us to take up the challenge of writing this book.

METHODS OF MANAGEMENT OF RELATIONSHIP TRIANGLES

Our approach to the clinical management of triangles is best summarized in the following five steps: (1) Find the triangle; (2) define the triangle's structure and the flow of movement within it; (3) reverse the flow of movement in the triangle; (4) expose the emotional process; (5) deal with the process and move toward improved functioning.

When Scott O. met Carolyn W. one summer on the beach, they were both 23. They were a year out of college, tired of the bar scene and the unending string of beer parties. Each of them had an unspoken longing to meet someone special who might turn out to be "the one." Neither of them believed that the chaotic madness of another Newport summer would provide the fulfillment of these wishes.

Now, 18 months later, Scott finds himself in a place he never dreamed he'd be: a psychiatrist's office. Scott and his family didn't really believe in psychiatry or "any of that mental health crap," but for the past 3 months Scott had been experiencing anxiety attacks at work, while driving to pick up Carolyn in the city, and even at a Giants' game with some old friends. The anxiety attacks included a pervasive sense of impending doom, with no rational stimulus, profuse sweating, heart palpitations, and nausea. All this in spite of the fact that his job was going well and his relationship with Carolyn was building in a beautiful way. In fact, in the past few months, especially around Christmas time, they had begun to talk about the possibility of becoming engaged on Carolyn's birthday in April.

Scott had consulted his family physician, concerned that he might have a cardiac problem. The physician had examined him and run the appropriate battery of tests, including an EKG and stress test, before telling Scott that he was physically fit and suffering from anxiety attacks. He prescribed small doses of Xanax, which gave Scott some relief. However, on a follow-up visit, Scott reported awakening at 3 A.M. each morning, in panic over the dream he was having that his mother was in a hospital with terminal cancer. In response to this information, the physician had referred Scott for a psychiatric evaluation.

The psychiatrist discontinued the Xanax and prescribed moderate doses of imipramine at bedtime. Imipramine is a tricyclic antidepressant with an excellent track record for controlling panic attacks. The psychiatrist assured Scott that his condition would respond to the medication if Scott complied with the treatment plan. He also asked some questions about Scott's life, looking for the developmental anxiety in him as well as the relationship processes that might be involved in the formation or maintenance of his symptoms.

Finding the Triangle

In Scott's case, the active triangle (Scott, his mother, and Carolyn) surrounding his anxiety symptoms was easy to see from the content of

Scott's dream and the developmental timing of the symptoms (just at the time his relationship with Carolyn was moving toward engagement). However, this clear presentation isn't the usual case: Finding triangles isn't always so easy. More likely someone like Scott would present his symptoms oblivious to their connections in time and relationship space. From shame, embarrassment, or denial, he would not mention his relationship with Carolyn or his repetitive dream about his mother, not seeing them as relevant. If the clinician Scott consulted thought only about biology, the treatment would consist only of prescribing an appropriate drug.

If the clinician believed in the importance of relationship process, his or her evaluation would include a search for developmental or situational issues in Scott's life. A logical focus would have been Scott's work and love life. Probes into either of these areas would have produced glowing reports from Scott. Only if the clinician had added a systems perspective to his knowledge of individuals and dyads would questions be directed toward potentially active relationship triangles in Scott's life.

For the fullest possible perspective on Scott, and to catch problems that might otherwise remain invisible, the clinician must be able to think about threes. Once the clinician does that it becomes simple, because the same tracks are followed to look for symptomatic triangles in any clinical case as are used to nail down individual and dyadic factors. The major tools in finding the relevant triangles are the patient's genogram and asking questions about the developmental and situational threats or challenges that are going on and about the triangles in the patient's relationship system that would most likely be activated. The genogram very quickly helps the clinician to visualize the developmental and situational challenges in the patient's life and so directs the flow of process questions. If Scott had presented clinically without making the key triangle explicit, these two sets of tools would do the trick.

But so what? In this case the imipramine would manage the symptoms well enough, and the panic attacks would go away. Scott would feel better and be none the worse off for lack of enlightenment about the cause of his anxiety. Clinically, one could defend this position, especially in light of the constraints of time and money and the demands for rapid symptom relief from our present models of care. This position can also be criticized, however. An equivalent, if a young patient presented to an internist with hypertension, would be for the internist to prescribe diuretics and other antihypertensive therapy without inquiring about family history, diet, and aerobic fitness.

In Scott's situation, even without the information about his marriage plans and dreams about his mother's death, a cursory look at the genogram would demonstrate the developmental challenges. A few well-placed process questions would uncover the active triangle. Process questions are formed more easily if you already have in your head a picture of possible triangles. With Scott, his mother, and Carolyn in mind, for example, some process questions might be: "How does your Mom like Carolyn?" "Did your mother have health problems or any separation anxiety when you or your sister left for college?" "How do you think your mother would do if you and Carolyn got married and your company transferred you to Europe?" "Does Carolyn admire the closeness you have with your mother?" "Does she worry about the impact that closeness might have on your marriage?"

Now, depending on how open Scott would have been to this type of questioning, his answers still might not yield much more information than you already had. Even as our society reels through this age of disclosure, psychiatry is being pushed by the edicts of managed care. After decades of probing to uncover internal and relationship conflicts, therapy has entered an age of containment. Even in the midst of this revolution, though, there remains a place for clinical discernment. Sound clinical judgment calls for at least a modest attempt to cut through denial rather than celebrate the superficial accounts of some patients by accepting their limited perspective and allowing it to dictate the course of treatment. It's worth the effort to take time to look for triangles.

Defining the Triangle's Structure and the Flow of Movement within It

Earlier in the book[1] we spoke of the difference between a relationship threesome and a relationship triangle. If we track the central triangle in Scott's life (with Carolyn and his mother) from the time he met Carolyn through the triangle's activation, we'd assume that the potential for an active triangle existed from the start. As Scott's relationship with Carolyn developed over time, the direction and intensity of his movement were increasingly toward Carolyn and away from his mother. It may have been that when Mrs. O. met Carolyn, in spite of

---

[1]See Chapter 3 (pp. 46–50).

feeling positive about her and pleasure in her instinctive feeling that Carolyn was the one for Scott, she found herself involuntarily asking Scott critical questions about Carolyn and their relationship. At this point the triangle was activated. Its structure, and the flow of movement in it, were largely determined by Scott's developmental challenge to separate from his mother and form a new primary relationship. Scott and Carolyn are closer in relation to one another, and Scott's mother is on the outside of their twosome.

There are many variations on this theme that could have occurred. Mrs. O. and Carolyn might have taken to each other and spoken so glowingly about each other to Scott that he might have become uncomfortable and started to wonder if he were doing the right thing. Or, their immediate appreciation of each other might have relieved Scott, as he felt Carolyn taking on the pressure of his relationship with his mother, and vice versa. In that case he might have come to believe that he was now relieved of obligations and free to spend time with his buddies without worrying about demands or criticism from either one of them. In fact, what happened was that Mrs. O. reacted with coolness toward Carolyn and was distant and critical (very much like Maureen O'Hara's character in the movie *Only the Lonely*). Carolyn responded by insisting that Scott get his mother under control and that he defend her against his mother or even that he choose between her or his mother.

The point is that, no matter what the variation, the problem Scott presents clinically will not be resolved successfully unless it's seen in triangular, as well as biological, individual, and dyadic terms. The underlying triangular process is the same whatever form the structure and movement take. It has to do with Scott separating from his mother and forming a new primary relationship: All three twosomes are interconnected and have to be dealt with—both separately and in their interconnectedness. Every new relationship in a person's life is affected by existing relationships. If the new relationship is (or should be) a primary one, it sets up the likelihood of conflicts about the primacy of attachment and the hierarchy of influence between the new relationship and the old ones.

Reversing the Flow of Movement

Once the therapist has a clear idea of the structure and the way the movement flows back and forth within the triangle, the first task is to create an experiment that reverses the direction of the relationship movement. Essentially, such experiments attempt to engage one or more members of the system to stop moving in the direction called for by affect and reactivity and to begin moving in a planned, experimental direction that usually is the opposite of what's been going on.

There are several reasons for doing this. First, the intervention increases self-focus, as people become aware of how difficult it is to do an apparently simple experiment in relationship movement. They begin to see themselves as caught and controlled by their emotions. Second, it gives people the sense that they have options in their behavior. There *are* ways of doing things differently from what they've been doing, which hasn't been working. Third, people's reactions to doing (or even thinking of doing) something different bring the underlying emotional process into the open.

The medication in the current case relieved Scott's panic attacks and took the edge off his inner turmoil. The psychiatrist offered him the option of accepting this as the result of treatment or of moving on to deal with the source of the anxiety that was driving his symptoms. Scott decided on the latter. Rather than deliver a lesson on triangles this early in therapy, which often creates confusion and misuse of the concept, the therapist suggested a relationship experiment. He pointed out to Scott that this was just that—an experiment, not necessarily a solution. While doing it, Scott was to monitor his own internal emotional reactions as well as the response in the relationship where the experiment is taking place.

He suggested that Scott move toward his mother (the opposite of what he had been doing). He suggested that Scott ask her what she thought about his closeness to Carolyn and the strong possibility that they might marry. Scott could open up with his mother the feelings he was having about not being so close to her any more and talk to her about how they could stay connected in ways appropriate for a mother and her married son. Scott could also just spend some relationship time with his mother, hanging out with her and talking about old times.

By this time, Carolyn had joined the therapy, and the therapist asked her, too, to perform an experiment. He predicted that she would have an emotional reaction of some kind to Scott's moves toward his mother, and he asked her to monitor it carefully. He suggested she might want to keep a journal of her reactions and bring it into the therapy. Carolyn did raise objections to Scott's spending more time with his mother, saying that Mrs. O. was against her and the marriage. The therapist pointed out that unless this triangle were resolved in some way, it would remain a permanent threat to their marriage. He said that Scott was doing the experiment for them and for the long-term health of their relationship, not for his mother.

The goal of Scott's experiment was to face his phobic avoidance of this mother, her understandable anxiety over losing her son, and the effect her anxiety had on him. The therapist offered two choices. One was for Scott to move directly toward his mother and spend some relationship time with her. Eventually he would talk to her about his anxiety, his symptoms, his plans with Carolyn, even about his and his mother's special relationship, and how they were going to deal with this difficult time in their lives.

A second option was for Scott to move toward his father and to discuss with him how to deal with his relationship problem with his mother. At first glance this option might appear to the novice triangle doctor as the activation of another triangle. But remember the distinction we made earlier between threesomes and triangles, we pointed out that behavior in an active triangle is driven by emotional reactivity. If Scott is moving toward his father to return the gift of his mother many years later, it's a developmentally appropriate, thoughtful, planned behavior. (Of course, if Scott's movement were laden with reactive feelings of anger and resentment toward his father, it would in fact represent the reactivation of Scott's primary parental triangle.)

At this point you may be thinking, "Well, if men are from Mars and women are from Venus, the families you see must be from Pluto if you can get them to do an experiment like moving toward either of their parents." This thinking raises the issue of clinical judgment: Which families and family members are coachable, and which will require the direct intervention of getting everyone into the treatment room? In general, coaching as a technique requires highly motivated, high-functioning adults with significant relationship leverage in their families. It also requires a belief that, through the modulation of anxiety and affect, and by means of relationship experiments, people's behavior in relationships can change. In the absence of some of these characteristics, it can still be useful to attempt coaching a patient through a relationship experiment. If coaching fails, then you can resort to enlarging the membership in the sessions to deal directly with the triangle.

In the meantime, let's return to Scott and his dilemma.

Exposing the Emotional Process in the Triangle

Six weeks later, after two more therapy sessions and a cancellation, Scott had yet to move toward his mother. Discussion with Scott uncovered his apprehension and aversion toward making this move. He also revealed that, in talking about this experiment with Carolyn, she kept saying she didn't get it. She thought that grown-ups drew boundaries between themselves and their parents. This was the reason she had moved from Baltimore to Connecticut and kept her visits home to a minimum.

The therapist repeated his earlier point that Scott didn't have to engage in the experiment. He could just take his medication and forget the project with his mother. However, he also offered Scott a plan to help him make up his mind about how to proceed. He lent him a video copy of *Only the Lonely,* a John Candy film about the struggle of a single Chicago cop who lived with his mother to separate from her and marry the woman of his dreams. The therapist suggested that Scott watch the tape with Carolyn and invite her to the next therapy session.

One of the purposes of a relationship experiment is to bring underlying emotional process to the surface. Just proposing this relationship experiment had revealed the following pieces of process:

1. Scott had an intense relationship with his mother and an inability to open up for discussion between them important issues in his and his mother's life. This lack of openness had forced the anxiety about these issues underground. The anxiety then came out by triggering Scott's biological vulnerability to panic attacks.

2. From his experience over the years, Scott had grave doubts about whether his father could or would be a supportive refuge for his mother as she suffered through the separation from Scott. In addition, his relationship with his father was weak enough that Scott couldn't ask his father to provide this support.

3. In his apprehension about the experiment, Scott's anxiety had been elevated, with two important side effects. First, there had been a moderate return of his panic symptoms. Second, a therapy triangle had been activated, consisting of Scott, Carolyn, and Scott's therapist.

It became the therapist's job to establish a plan to neutralize this threefold process.

Neutralizing the Process and Detriangling

The therapist had begun Scott's treatment by managing his symptoms of anxiety and then moving on to assist him in addressing the symptomatic triangle with Carolyn and his mother. The relationship experiment, designed with this triangle in mind, did its job by opening up the process described above: Scott's anxious attachment to his mother and his inability to communicate with her about difficult issues; his insufficient attachment to his father; the formation of a therapy triangle around the experiment.

The activation of a therapy triangle almost always calls for dealing with it immediately. Scott's taking *Only the Lonely* home to watch with Carolyn was the first of a number of steps designed to involve her in the therapy. Perhaps now is a good time to raise a philosophical (and perhaps ethical) question about the methods we're describing. Someone who adheres to a minimalist approach to therapy might argue that all this playing around with Scott's triangles is producing iatrogenic problems—not to mention prolonging the therapy and increasing its cost. Such a critic might add that, if Scott's panic attacks had failed to respond to medication and cognitive techniques, or that, if after initial relief he had suffered multiple relapses, the treatment described here could be offered as an adjunct to fortify the primary intervention. However, we believe in a heavy emphasis on patient education and efforts at prevention. Primary care medicine today emphasizes the importance of changes in diet, exercise, and life style in caring for cardiac- and cancer-prone patients. In much the same way, we believe that work on relationship triangles is essential to the comprehensive care of anxiety, depression, and relationship conflict. It's important to educate patients about the choices available to them for elective procedures and to allow them to make a choice.

We return now to Scott and his fiancee. Carolyn came to the next session and, in a clear and forthright way, gave her thoughts on Scott's situation. She said that they had both enjoyed *Only the Lonely* and after watching it had a long discussion about driving to Baltimore so that Scott could meet her family. They saw this as a step on the road to getting engaged. At that point, the therapist asked Carolyn about her family and how it differed from Scott's. He also asked her directly if she thought the separation between Scott and his mother might go better by dealing openly with the issues between them rather than leaving them unspoken and having everyone anxious about them. Carolyn said that she could imagine it but had never seen it work. The therapist asked her to help him by trying to get emotionally neutral about the idea and by sitting back and evaluating the results with him. He added that, with Scott's and his parents' permission, he would videotape the sessions and allow her to study them as a part of her evaluation. If she liked the results, she might even get Scott to take the camcorder along to on the trip to Baltimore.

Carolyn expressed the thought that the therapist was even more relentless than her mother, but she agreed to the challenge. Scott agreed to speak with his parents about coming in for a series of three sessions to deal with some issues that were important to him.

All these steps were aimed at neutralizing the therapy triangle that the proposed experiment had activated. The therapist depolarized the triangle by decreasing the distance between him and Carolyn, thereby diminishing the emotional reactivity in the therapy triangle. If the therapist had tried to bring Carolyn in to lecture her on how she was blocking Scott's therapy, to convert her to the therapist's way of thinking, or to shut her out of the work Scott would do with his parents, the triangle would have gotten further polarized and reactive. Therapy might in fact be dead in the water for the foreseeable future.

The therapist hoped that, in addition to neutralizing the therapy triangle, by his engaging Carolyn actively in the process, other good things would happen. If Scott and his parents were successful, enough of a conversion would take place in Carolyn that she would support the present therapeutic efforts and that the potential for future problems (or at least the fallout from future problems) would be diminished.

With the therapy triangle under control, the work with Scott and his parents could begin. Scott's reluctance when the experiment had been suggested made it clear that coaching him was unlikely to work. Directly involving his parents in therapy seemed the most efficient way to deal with Scott's overly strong attachment to his mother and his weak attachment to his father. The feelings of loss that go along with kids growing up are as predictable as the moon and tides, but they're usually handled by angry distance or silent emotional paralysis. The first item on the agenda, therefore, was making it safe enough for Scott and his mother to talk about the emotional side of their developmental problems.

To make the therapy "safe," the therapist's questions in the first session gently and curiously addressed the family's ability to deal with the hard feelings (anger and resentment) versus the tender feelings (loss and longing). Scott and his mother did most of the talking about this in the first session, and they planned to continue doing so outside the therapy. (It might seem that encouraging all this talking and connection between Scott and his mother intensifies and prolongs the separation difficulties. Our experience and our theory predict just the opposite: it's the *failure* to communicate openly and work through these overly close connections that makes separation more of a problem.)

In the second session, the therapist directed the discussion toward the question of whether either side of the family had a tradition of the men being connected to one another in a way that was emotionally supportive. The idea was to plant a seed that might germinate and foster an improvement in the attachment between Scott and his father.

In the third session, the therapist asked Scott's father for his opinion about the first two sessions. Mr. O. said he thought they'd been worthwhile; he hoped his son thought so, too. About 15 minutes into this session, Mrs. O. somewhat hesitantly said that the first two sessions brought up for her the topic of *her own* mother-in-law. She said she hadn't wanted to talk about it then but asked her husband if he would come back to the therapist with her and without Scott to talk about Mr. O.'s relationship with his mother and the impact that relationship had had on her. Mr. O. looked thunderstruck and said that he wasn't sure what his wife was talking about. He agreed reluctantly to a session with her, but he had great difficulty settling on an appointment time.

Carolyn came in one more time with Scott. She had watched one of the tapes of the sessions with Scott's parents and said that it looked too good to be true but that she'd be willing to keep an open mind. She kidded the therapist about bringing him along on the trip to Baltimore. No further appointments were scheduled, and the therapist told Scott to call if he wanted to do some more work or if his anxiety symptoms returned.

The follow-up of treatment proved satisfactory. With the help of the imipramine, Scott hadn't had a recurrence of panic attacks for 6 months. When the psychiatrist saw him at that time, he explained that there were two options—to taper off the medicine, or to remain on a maintenance dose for a longer time. Scott asked the psychiatrist to write down the schedule for tapering off, and made a follow-up appointment. He cancelled that appointment, and the psychiatrist didn't hear from Scott, Carolyn, or Scott's parents for 4 years. At that time, Scott called for an appointment. Just the day before, on the train going to work, he had experienced another panic attack. So, he thought he ought to check with the therapist before the situation got out of hand. When he came in, Scott reported that he and Carolyn had been married for 2½ years and were very happy. He also said that things were going well with his mother—she and Carolyn had been getting along fine, and he had been careful to maintain a relationship with his mother. As the session neared its close, the therapist remained puzzled that he could find no trigger for the panic attack Scott reported. On his way out the door, after making an appointment for a few weeks later, Scott smiled and said, "By the way, Doc, we just found out 2 weeks ago that Carolyn is pregnant."

SUMMARY AND CONCLUSION

This chapter has reviewed the pervasiveness of relationship triangles in people's lives, both personal and professional. Scott's developmental struggle illustrates the part triangles play in the predictable events of all our lives.

All therapists, whatever their theoretical persuasions, have listened to Scott's story and ones like it repeatedly in their offices. In their personal lives, therapists have experienced triangles activated by the birth of a baby, the death of a parent, a child leaving home for college. Our purpose has been to make you, the reader, a "triangle doctor." This chapter, therefore, together with the rest of the book, gives you the tools to do that. We've given you a developmental history of the concept of relationship triangles. We've analyzed the idea by breaking it down into its component parts: structure, movement, process, and function. To make it easier to use triangles in clinical work, we've offered a clinical typology of the most-often-seen triangles and a clinical methodology for dealing with them. We've presented information that leads to knowledge and recognition of triangles. We've shown how triangles set up structurally, how emotional process flows through the structure, and how triangles serve functions for any relationship system.

In order to make a working knowledge of triangles more useful clinically, we proposed our five-step paradigm in this chapter. This method allows for identifying the triangles that people bring to us and the ones that we create in therapy and in our own lives, for understanding them, and for intervening with them. Now, using the genogram to grasp the context of the individual's or the dyad's symptoms, and with the topology of triangles in your head, you can *find* the triangle or triangles that you need to work on. Having done that, you can now *define the structure* of the triangle and *see the flow of movement* in it. Once you're clear about structure and movement, you can then begin to intervene by *reversing the flow of movement* experimentally. If people follow your suggestion and do the experiment, inevitably that will *expose the emotional process* that has been hiding underneath the symptoms. The experiment will expose the emotional process to you and to the individual, couple, or family, and now you can *deal with it* directly and move people toward improved functioning.

It is our firm belief, based on years of experience, that developing a radar for spotting triangles gives therapists a wider perspective on possible interventions for every case they see. This can't help but positively affect clinical outcomes.

In closing, we'd like to reemphasize a point essential to good clinical practice. to work skillfully in triangles, a therapist must also be skilled at working with individuals and dyads. As the practice of psychotherapy evolves over time and cost-effectiveness becomes more of a factor in therapy, it's important to develop the ability to integrate the following three factors: (1) the biological and psychological pro-cesses internal to the individual, (2) the emotional processes in relationship dyads that gives those individuals the important connections in their lives, and (3) the inevitable reactive emotional triangles that are an integral part of relationships and form the essential building blocks of any relationship system. Effective psychotherapy relieves symptoms, opens the door to and facilitates the process of psychological change for individuals, and improves the nature of the connections with one another. The fabric of this therapy is woven out of an integration of individual, dyadic, and triangular factors. In fact, you could say that this is the one-two-three of psychotherapy.

References

American Psychiatric Association. 1994. *Diagnostic and Statistical Manual of Mental Disorders, Fourth Edition (DSM-IV)*. Washington, DC: American Psychiatric Association.

Bowen, Murray. 1957. *Treatment of Family Groups with a Schizophrenic Member*. Paper presented at the annual meeting of the American Orthopsychiatric Association, Chicago.

Bowen, Murray. 1966. "The Use of Family Theory in Clinical Practice." *Comprehensive Psychiatry, 7,* 345–374.

Bowen, Murray, 1978a. *Family Therapy in Clinical Practice*. New York: Jason Aronson.

Fogarty, Thomas. 1975. "Triangles." *The Family, 2,* 11–20.

Fogarty, Thomas. 1979. "The Distancer and the Pursuer." *The Family, 7*(1), 11–16.

Freud, Sigmund. 1955 (1913). "Totem and Taboo." In *The Standard Edition of the Complete Psychological Works of Sigmund Freud, Volume 14*. London: Hogarth Press and the Institute of Psycho-analysis.

Guerin, Philip, Leo Fay, Susan Burden, and Judith Kautto. 1987. *The Evaluation and Treatment of Marital Conflict*. New York: Basic Books.

Guerin, Philip, and Edward Gordon. 1986. "Trees, Triangles and Temperament in the Child-Centered Family." In *Evolving Models for Family Change: A Volume in Honor of Salvador Minuchin*, Eds. H. Charles Fishman and Bernice L. Rosman. New York: Guilford Press.

Haley, Jay. 1987. *Problem-Solving Therapy, Second Edition*. San Francisco: Jossey-Bass.

Kerr, Michael, and Murray Bowen. 1988. *Family Evaluation*. New York: Norton.

Luepnitz, Deborah Anna. 1988. *The Family Interpreted: Feminist Theory in Clinical Practice*. New York: Basic Books.

Minuchin, Salvador. 1974. *Families and Family Therapy.* Cambridge, MA: Harvard University Press.

Pittman, Frank. 1989. *Private Lies: Infidelity and the Betrayal of Intimacy.* New York: Norton.

Speck, Ross V., and Carolyn L. Attneave. 1973. *Family Networks.* New York: Pantheon.

Index